I0438827

BLUNDERS IN THE KITCHEN

Diet Mistakes to Avoid While Fueling the
Perfect Beach Physique

By Marshall A. Nash

Legal Notice and Disclaimer:

This publication is designed to provide competent and reliable information regarding the subject matter covered. However, it was written for informational and entertainment purposes only. It is sold with the understanding that the author and publisher are not engaged in professional advice, but rather the author is merely providing opinions and beliefs based on personal experiences and first-hand knowledge as a personal fitness trainer and nutritional coach. It is the author's belief that the information provided is accurate, but the author and publisher specifically disclaim any liability that may be incurred from the use or application of the contents of this book. Always seek the advice of your physician before beginning any exercise and or nutritional plan.

Cover art by: Christopher Godsoe

Edited by: Nathan Chamberlain

Interior design by: Marshall Nash

First Edition: July 2017. Blunders Series: 2

Library of Congress Control Number: 2017910282

CreateSpace Independent Publishing Platform, North Charleston, SC

ISBN: 9781548378066

Printed in the United States of America

For Kenzie and Mikie

Acknowledgements:

I would like to say thank you for all the support to my family, friends, and fans. Writing this book has been a rewarding endeavor. It's been a blessing to be able to share my knowledge of a subject I am abundantly passionate about. I would like to give a special thank you to my best pal Riff Johnson. A vast amount of the knowledge I have gathered on food that is contained in this book was originally obtained through counsel from my lifelong friend Riff. All the information I have ever received that is included in this book has been confirmed by my own personal, diligent research, but much of it has originated from other knowledgeable family members and friends, whom I thank dearly.

I also want to give a special thank you to my cousin Jennifer Brawn, who has been very helpful in providing me a vast amount of valuable information on different foods and diet that I was previously unaware of. A special thank you is in order for my fellow author and brother Nathan Chamberlain for his steadfast and amazing editing work on this book. Thank you, Nate, without your help, many flaws may not have come to light, so I thank you. Also, a special thank you has been earned for my good friend and another fellow author Christopher Godsoe for his incredible artwork in designing the cover for this book. You are multi-talented, my friend.

I want to say a special thank you as well for your support and many years of friendship to both Scott and Jay Downing (Ice Cream Man and Pudding Boy respectfully.) My pals Scott and Jay are known by their nicknames for two of my favorite cheat foods. Hey, life does allow enjoyment of some fine treats now and again. Life would be a bore if we couldn't occasionally indulge in a cheat and still look and feel like a million bucks! It has been said many times that no man is an island. There is much truth to this statement. I could not have produced the kind of book I have to present to you without the help and support of others, so thank you very much; this book is made possible by your advice and labor too.

Contents

Introduction: *Stay in the Kitchen and Take the Heat!*

I love food. Anyone who knows me can attest to this. My strong love for food has made achieving the body of my dreams an incredible challenge over the years. It's been a huge obstacle I've had to learn how to overcome in order to reach my health and fitness goals. However, food was not always such a vice for me. When I was a kid, I was a scrawny little pipsqueak who barely ate. Boy, did that change over the years. I remember when I was a young boy, it was quite the task to get me to stop running around and playing just to sit down and have a bite to eat; unless it was a sugar filled treat (my sweet tooth has been something of a legend). Four teeth pulled, and three root canals later have forced me to take a seriously hard look at my sugar addiction.

As I grew up into adulthood, my appetite grew right alongside me. As of now, at 37 years old as of this writing, I've gone from extremely skinny, to a pile of pudge, and back again. I've done this feat on more than one occasion, believe it or not. Unlike my no-appetite pipsqueak days, adulthood has been a different story of a ravenous appetite. Except during my younger years, I've always struggled with diet. Through this challenge, I've experienced every kind of diet blunder you could imagine. I've always been into fitness, but it wasn't until I was much older (in my 30's, actually) that I indeed learned that you cannot just eat whatever you want just because you work out. You cannot produce a ripped, beach physique this way. Due to my obsession to get a ripped and shredded body, I was forced to learn the hard way on how to truly eat the right way by making diet blunder after diet blunder and learning from my countless mistakes.

All of my negative experiences with dieting, along with intense, personal research, and my formal education as a nationally certified personal fitness trainer has enabled me to compile all of the do's and don'ts you will ever need in order to eat the right way and achieve the body of your dreams. I wrote this book to give you the advice you need to not only achieve the body of your dreams through the diet part of the diet/exercise factors, but also to help you be healthier, lose weight, and maintain a healthy weight. The information in this book when applied will help you to achieve that overall damn good feeling you have when you are healthy and enjoy a better quality of life because of it. I want that for everyone. I love helping people. The mission I have for this book is to reach as many individuals in the world as I possibly can to help them have the knowledge of what diet mistakes you need to avoid, and what you need to be doing in place of all those possible diet blunders. My mission, if successful, can help you live life with remarkably good health, feel like a million bucks, and live the best quality of life you possibly can. This is my hope of what this book can do for you.

Some of what is contained in this book might be considered common sense, but I think it's good to be refreshed on the basics of dieting from time to time. It's important to be reminded of what the best things are that you can be doing with your diet, and what you need to be avoiding. This book isn't about any one particular kind of diet. You will not find any "fad" or special kind of diet here as I believe those are mostly a waste of time. What you will find in this book is how to achieve and attain nutritional balance, how to avoid detrimental diet mistakes, and what diet habits and rules to follow for your best health, and physique. Use this book as your nutritional guide. Some things in this book are not common sense at all; some of it is scientific, some of it is motivational, but as a whole, it's all you'll ever need to know about the rules of successful dieting.

Chapter One: *Big Mac, Little Fella*

Lesson 1: Volume of food is a top priority in dieting.

Okay, so we all know we shouldn't gorge our faces until we can hardly breathe. However, even this most basic rule in dieting needs to be refreshed in our minds from time to time to remind ourselves to avoid this detrimental habit, and replace it with healthy habits. Overeating is probably the most common kitchen blunder most people make, including myself. I have been very guilty of this in the past. I've eaten many meals that after the last bite I would end up eating so much that I'd look extremely bloated and my breathing would be noticeably affected. Overeating can become a very destructive habit that leads to you guessed it, more overeating. Not only that, but you can literally make the size of your stomach much bigger than normal just by overeating.[1]

Your stomach will adapt to the volume of food you put in it.[1] Eat tiny amounts, and it will shrink, which will ordinarily make you feel fuller with only small amounts of food. On the flip side to that coin, shovel a boatload of hotdogs down the grocery hole as if you're in some crazy eating contest, and your stomach will have the opposite effect; your stomach will expand, even massively if you shovel too much down in there too often. So how should we go about curbing this blunder?

You have to always be mindful of how much you are actually eating during the entire course of each meal. Never underestimate the importance of doing this. Part of the reason for this is that it can take roughly 20 minutes before your brain will tell you, oh yeah, your stomach is full; you don't need to keep eating![2] If you're plopped down on the couch and just gorging away being all distracted, then you could very easily overeat, especially with snacks like chips, for example. If you're not truly staying mindful of what you are putting in your mouth at all times, before you know it you have woofed down half that bag of chips, or crackers, or hell maybe even half a jug of ice cream, or pudding maybe? Either way, whatever it is you're snacking on it could very easily end up being too much, even if it's a healthy snack; too much of something like peanut butter could be fattening.

The best thing that I recommend you do is always to portion out how much you are going to eat before every meal or snack time. Once the portions are gone, the snack or meal is over. Keep more of that food, or any food, out of sight. Put it in the fridge, the cupboard, or wherever it belongs. That way you can't just say that it won't matter if I just grab a little bit more here that's just sitting on the table, or on the stand next to the couch while snacking during the game, TV show, or what have you. Now you don't need to eat like a bird and portion out two tiny pieces of food on your dish, but you don't want it overflowing on the rim either.

Another tactic you can use to curb overeating is to drink plenty of water before and during a meal or snack time. Drinking some water will help you feel full without having to consume as much food to get that fullness feeling.[1] I recommend drinking at least a glass full of water before your meal and keep sipping on some while you're eating as well. Finally, using containers and measuring out how much you need for all your food groups for each meal or snack is one of the best strategies you can utilize to combat overeating. Do this, and you'll be developing a positive habit that will benefit you greatly in your dieting.

Chapter One Summary:

- **Be mindful of how much you are eating during each meal/snack. Avoiding overeating is imperative to dieting success.**

- **Stomach size will adapt to the volume of food you feed it, which will affect how much food will make you feel full.**

- **The best strategy to avoid overeating is to portion out all meals/snacks before eating.**

- **Ideally, you should use containers to measure out your portions for each food group every single day.**

Chapter Two: *Too Little, or Too Much?*

Lesson 2: It's better to eat many small meals throughout the day rather than a few big ones.

One of the greatest mistakes I see many individuals make when they are on a mission to lose weight is that they hardly eat. I can't count how many times I've heard someone say they only eat once or twice a day. Folks, this is wrong on so many levels. This will not help you lose weight and keep it off. This is not healthy. This is counterproductive. Don't do this. Also, the standard American three square meals a day is so far outdated. Science now tells us this is not the best way to feed our bodies. It's not the best way for weight control, or to control steady blood sugar levels.[3]

The best way to keep your energy levels the most stable, and blood sugar relatively even, is to eat five small meals a day rather than three big ones.[3] You should be eating about every three hours or so. It should go like this: breakfast, snack, lunch, snack, then supper, rest and repeat the next day. One meal that's often skipped, which shortens the number of meals in a day is breakfast.

Skipping breakfast is a big no-no. Doing this once in a while won't necessarily result in a significant setback with your diet goals, but I don't recommend you do this often. Skipping breakfast or a meal once in a while can give your digestive system a small break and may even have some benefits to it,[4] but don't do this excessively; maybe once or twice a month if you choose to. Eating breakfast is vital if you want to have success in your dieting for many reasons.

Eating breakfast helps to kick start your metabolism for the day.[3] You want your metabolism revved up for the better part of the day to burn the most fuel. Not only that, but it will help make you feel more energetic if you eat healthy foods for breakfast. Who doesn't want more energy during the day, especially in the morning when you're first trying to get going? On top of that, skipping breakfast can lead to a gorge fest later on. When you finally decide to eat after skipping breakfast, it's easy to overcompensate due to the fact you've been running on empty for a lengthy amount of time (especially when considering you're not consuming any food the entire time you sleep through the night.) More times than not this is what will end up happening. Now breakfast doesn't have to be huge. In fact, I don't recommend a large breakfast. You want to kick start your metabolism into high gear, but eat too much food and you run the risk of feeling bogged down. You will end up feeling heavy and won't feel awake like you want to first thing in the morning.

I recommend a good sized breakfast, but contrary to popular belief it should not be your biggest meal.[3] Lunch should be your biggest meal, breakfast second in size, and dinner should be your smallest meal in the day.[3] Usually, what happens though is just the opposite. Many simply skip breakfast. Lunch is a medium size meal for most people, and then later in the day at dinner time when you require the least amount of food for energy is when people tend to go the heaviest.

Dinner time being the biggest meal is what happens in a lot of cases, and for many, bedtime doesn't fall too far behind supper. I know for many people their work schedules make timing dinner, or almost any meal, very challenging, but you have to try and do your very best with this. Plan out your meals for the day ahead of time the best you possibly can. Any amount of time saved by favorable planning is a plus.

Chapter Two Summary:

- **The standard three square meals a day is outdated and should be replaced with five small meals throughout the day.**

- **Eating every few hours helps to keep your energy and blood sugar levels more stable.**

- **Rarely skip breakfast. When you take the time to eat breakfast you are jump starting your metabolism. Eating breakfast can help prevent a gorge fest later on when you're feeling the effects of a stomach** running on empty for a lengthy amount of time. A once in a while break for your digestive system by skipping breakfast or any other meal is ok, as long as you don't do this excessively.

- Contrary to popular belief, breakfast should NOT be your biggest meal. Lunch should be biggest, breakfast second largest, dinner and snacks in between meals should be the smallest.

- Meal planning can be difficult with a hectic and busy schedule, but do your best to make it a habit of planning out all meals. This can save time and is a positive diet habit.

Chapter Three: *All Calories Are Not Created Equal!*

Lesson 3: The cliché "a calorie is a calorie is a calorie" is a lie!

I think if whoever made up this ridiculous term was forced to go on an all-sugar diet to test this theory, "a calorie is a calorie is a calorie" and see what it does to their body and health; then I think they would never say this term again. Can we please kill this statement once and for all!? This statement couldn't be further from the truth, and it is so misleading to anyone trying to diet correctly; especially when trying to lose weight. It's almost like saying, "hey just go right ahead and stuff your face with whatever foods you desire. As long as it's under a certain number of calories than it won't cause any harm. Oh, and you can still lose weight." If you value your health and trying to lose weight, I plead with you to never heed this moronic advice.

However, I will admit there is certainly some truth to the fact that the number of calories consumed is directly linked to your weight, and when it comes to weight loss, the fewer calories you take in, compared to those you burn, will naturally increase weight loss; except in rare cases where a medical condition could be inhibiting your ability to lose weight. In truth, calories do not lie; calories are unforgiving. Either you ate that cupcake, or you didn't. However, for anyone to suggest that all calories are equal is outright crazy. If any dieticians still use this term, they should be either retrained or fired. The term that should be utilized in its place should be better quality calories, better healthier body.

What you put in your body is incredibly important and can have both positive and negative effects that extend far beyond the calorie content of the food you consume. Look at it this way; if you were to eat nothing but ice cream all day, but your intake remained at 2,000 calories, it would not be equal to eating 2,000 calories worth of vegetables. How do you think you would feel at the end of the day if you chose the first option over the latter? With the veggies, I think you would agree that you are putting in far better quality calories as opposed to what you get with the ice cream option. Would you agree that if all you ate was ice cream, chances are you'd end up looking pretty flabby? Would you also agree that if all you ate was vegetables, even though that's not necessarily a balanced diet, it's going to make you feel better and look thinner than if all you ate was ice cream? I think most of us would agree with that.

Besides that, how much food is 2,000 calories worth of ice cream? A couple bowls full? You are going to feel much fuller with the fiber filled, quality energy giving vegetables than you are with a relatively small amount of sugary goodness from the ice cream that will only give you a temporary sugar rush. Remember, a diet of sugar will lead to a sugar high, but then a crash, which will only leave you hungry again in a short amount of time! These two different foods are not going to make you feel the same way, and they certainly won't have the same effect on your body. I think it's safe to say that is just some plain common sense, and this common sense will serve you well. Another way to put it is to think of food as fuel. With the right fuel, your body can have the ability to operate at peak efficiency. You must have the right fuel. Think of your body working like a car does. A car needs gas to run, but it needs quality gas to run its best. If you mix some water or dirt in your gas, it won't run right. It will still run, but it most certainly will not run right. Over time you can damage your car by giving it dirty gas as opposed to clean gas. It works the same way with food as fuel for your body.

Finally, anyone who still uses the term "a calorie is a calorie is a calorie," especially professionals, needs to stop and give that term some serious thought. A calorie is not a calorie is not a calorie! I tell you this because I want you to know that regardless of calorie content - not just how much you eat, but what you eat - absolutely matters.

Chapter Three Summary:

- **Don't listen to so-called gurus or professional dietitians who somehow still think "a calorie is a calorie is a calorie!"**

- **Given the same amount of calories when comparing a bowl of ice cream to the equivalent calorie content as eating vegetables, common sense tells us vegetables are the all-around better choice.**

- **There is truth to the fact that fewer calories in than out will result in weight loss if you don't have an underlying medical condition, but this does not mean just eat whatever you want as long as it's under a certain number of calories.**

- **Not just how much you eat, but the quality of, and what you eat, matters too.**

Chapter Four: *The Scale vs. the Mirror*

Lesson 4: Pay more attention to visual change rather than a number on a scale.

It is not psychologically beneficial for you to obsess over your weight and to step on the scale to check your weight every day.[5] When dieting and trying to lose weight, I can completely relate to how frustrating it can be to have to be patient to see results from your efforts. What I see a lot of times are people weighing themselves on a daily basis because they want that number on the scale to go down; they just can't wait for it to happen. The problem with this is the fact that your weight can fluctuate up or down a few pounds from day to day.[6] You can weigh yourself one day, and it appears you have lost a pound or two, but then you weigh yourself again the next day, and you've gained back those pounds; maybe even added another two! Even if you are following all the diet rules in this book and you're doing everything perfectly right, this can still happen; and it's completely normal. Ok, so what's going on that can make your weight fluctuate?

There are three main things in your body that can fluctuate daily which can sway your weight one way or the other. Water retention, bodily waste accumulation, and the food you have eaten during the day are the three things that can change on any given day, hence why your weight can fluctuate within a few pounds on a daily basis.[6] This is one reason why I caution you not to weigh yourself every day, no matter how tempting it is to see if you are getting any closer to your diet goals; whether it is to lose weight, or even to put on some weight.

It can be very upsetting mentally if you are doing well with your diet, trying to lose weight, when suddenly the scale jumps up for no apparent reason. This is exactly what can happen if you weigh yourself too often. You don't want to accidentally put yourself in panic mode without knowing that what's going on is perfectly normal. The scale isn't going to tell you exactly what's going on with your body. If you step on that scale every day, I can guarantee you that it's not always going to reveal that you're getting closer to your goals.

What I recommend, rather than weighing yourself every day, is to first pay attention to the mirror over anything else. The mirror doesn't lie; this is where you will see real change. You have to be extremely patient though because when you are doing things that can lead to long-lasting results, these body changes will appear very slowly, and they will be subtle. If you stick with the plan and diet correctly, you will see positive changes over time. That alone can feel extremely gratifying and, trust me, it is well worth the wait to get there. The mirror trumps the scale any given day of the week. Now, I don't recommend you completely ignore the scale, just don't obsess over the number. The mirror is *always* more important than a scale. Now, just checking your sexy self out in the mirror every day isn't giving you the whole picture. I do recommend that you use a scale occasionally because it does have its place, and it certainly does give you some useful information.

Rather than weighing yourself every single day, I recommend that you weigh yourself just once a week. And remember that your weight can fluctuate, so don't be alarmed if you don't always see a positive change towards your goals on the scale even if you only weigh yourself once a week. The trick is to look for the trend. Take a month and look at what's happened over that span of time, or any amount of time that you choose to gauge yourself with. If you were to plot your weight on a graph, it would tell you the trend, and you will see it with your very own eyes.

When looking at the trend of your weigh-ins, you need to ask yourself if your weight is going up, down, or staying relatively the same. It's perfectly reasonable if you were to look at a graph of your weight change and see some bumps in the road; remember weight fluctuates. The trend, along with the mirror, will tell you what you need to know. Also, it is better to use a body-fat analyzer if you have one, rather than just a weight scale, because losing body fat should be your true goal if you are aiming to lose weight. You can buy an inexpensive body-fat analyzer online. Some weight scales even have body-fat analyzers built right into them, which is a bonus. Now, the timing of when you choose to do your weigh-ins is important as well.

The best time to weigh yourself is first thing in the morning.[6] This should be after using the bathroom, with little or no clothing, and before you have eaten anything. Since we know that one of the fluctuating factors is whether or not your bladder or bowels are full, it only makes sense to weigh yourself after you have gone to the bathroom. Also, since what you have eaten, especially recently, is another weight fluctuating factor, the morning is the very best time to weigh yourself. Unless you are a sleep walker and you take a random trip to the fridge, your stomach should be relatively empty. This should certainly be true if you also followed the rule of not eating at least three hours before going to bed. We will touch on that rule later. Finally, weighing yourself in the nude or with little clothing means you won't be seeing the additional weight from your clothing on the scale.

You would be surprised how much clothing or shoes and boots will weigh if you were to weigh yourself with these on, and then take them off and re-weigh yourself. I guarantee you that the weight difference will be at least a couple of pounds. So, weighing yourself in the morning with little to no clothing, and after you have gone to the bathroom, is clearly going to give you the most accurate body weight measurement. By doing this you are eliminating, or at the very least reducing, some of the fluctuating factors that can give you a less than accurate (and higher) number on that pesky weight scale. The worst time to weigh yourself would be at night. By the end of the evening, you've accumulated all the food you've eaten during the day and chances are that your body has not had time to digest and eliminate all of it. If you are bloated, that could add to the number on the scale as well. So, now that you know that, how much is a good number of pounds to lose every week if you are trying to shed some pudge?

If weight loss is your goal, the ideal amount of weight that you should be losing every week is one to two pounds of fat.[7] This is the sweet spot of long-term weight loss. Anything more than one to two pounds per week is potentially too fast, and you could be doing more harm than good when looking at things long-term.[3] Quick results are not the best way to go. You should want to achieve those results in a way that is likely to be lasting, not temporary. Barring an overactive metabolism, if you are losing more than one to two pounds a week you are dieting too strictly, exercising too excessively, or a combination of both. If you're losing more than this, chances are you could be burning off an excessive amount of muscle in addition to fat, which is detrimental to the speed of your metabolism.[3]

The speed of your metabolism is directly affected by the amount of muscle you have.[8] So, naturally, the more muscle you have, the more efficient your body will be at burning calories throughout the day.[8] It takes far more energy for your body to cater to muscle than it does to fat.[9] The lower your body fat percentage, the higher the level your overall metabolism will operate at.[112] When you are dieting, it is typical to lose a small amount of muscle.[3] This is nearly unavoidable, but when it's excessive due to extreme behavior, it becomes troublesome. It's also important to point out that if you make any sudden changes to your diet, or if you start a new workout (especially one that is high intensity) then it may take a while before you notice much (if any) weight loss and changes.[112] This may sound strange, but there is a good explanation for this.

When you put a sudden stress on your body that it's not used to, your body may end up retaining water as a way of protecting itself against this sudden unknown stress.[112] I say this because if you suddenly change up your diet, or begin working out, don't be alarmed if you don't see any changes in your weight or body composition (which is the percentages of fat and fat free tissue in the body, which are the amount of muscle, organs, water, bone, and other tissues in your body)[10] right away. If your body goes into protection mode against a new stress, then it may take some time for your body to adapt and realize, oh hey! This is good for me! At that point, when your body wakes the hell up and realizes that you are putting good stress on it, that is when you should start to see some changes. If you do not see any changes after six weeks, I recommend checking with your doctor.[11]

If you are doing everything correctly, but no changes are happening after the first six weeks of starting a new diet or exercise regiment, it is possible you may have an underlying medical condition.[11] If you suspect that this may be the case, I highly recommend consulting with your doctor. If it appears to be impossible to lose any weight, it's not a bad idea to ask your doctor to check you for an underactive thyroid.[12] An underactive thyroid can cause your metabolism to operate very slowly. This can happen because the thyroid is a gland that helps to control your metabolism, so it's a good idea to get this checked if it seems to be impossible to lose weight.[13] The opposite of this can be true as well; if you have an overactive thyroid, it can be nearly impossible to gain weight.[112] A doctor can run tests that will tell you if your thyroid is behaving normally or not. I also want to point out that when you first start dieting and/or working out, you may experience a much higher rate of weight loss than the recommended one to two pounds a week, in the first few weeks.[112]

If your body doesn't react to a new diet or exercise regimen by holding onto water, then the exact opposite can happen. What happens in most cases is, rather than holding onto water, your body gets rid of excess water when you are first beginning to eat right or exercise.[112] This is both good and bad. It's good because before your body can start tapping into fat reserves that you want to go away, it first has to get rid of this excess water that your body doesn't need. The unfortunate part about this is the fact that when you start doing the things that are conducive to lose weight (dieting and/or exercising more), it's hard not to get overexcited when weighing yourself after the first week and think, *wow I've lost six pounds!* I caution you not to get overexcited here. It's great that your overall body weight is suddenly going in the direction you want it to go in, but be mindful that this much weight loss in a short amount of time means it is more than likely it's not all fat that's been lost, but mostly water.[112] Will some of it be fat? That is very possible. Just keep in mind that for the first few weeks you definitely could be seeing more than one to two pounds of weight loss. However, don't be disappointed after the first few weeks if your weight loss goes from being high to just the average one to two pounds a week. Know that this is a good thing! This means that your body is now getting rid of the stuff you don't want; fat! This is the kind of weight loss you want, but you certainly don't want to be burning off muscle.

The way to avoid your body from using muscle as energy when you really want to be losing fat is to make sure you are not too strict with your diet. I see this mistake so often; eating like a bird when what you really need to eat like is a human. Eating too little is what can cause your body to begin using muscle instead of fat for energy when trying to lose weight.[14] Now, why would your body do this if you're borderline starving yourself? You see, the body is this wonderfully operating creation that has its own best interest at hand; to protect itself. This all goes back to the stress that I was talking about before. What happens when you are barely eating anything, instead of losing fat, is that your body will go into starvation mode. In starvation mode, your body wants to protect itself by holding onto body fat that it thinks it will need later on.[14] You can't just tell your body what you want it to burn off for energy. How wonderful it would be if only it worked that way, but it doesn't, so you have to eat!

What frequently happens in cases where someone has been borderline starving themselves is that they do end up losing a bunch of weight, but it's not sustainable. This is because they have lost too much muscle along with some fat. Because of this muscle loss, their metabolism has slowed down to a state slower than before - maybe even to a crawl.[112] As soon as you start eating normally again, your body will burn fewer calories than before. This slower metabolism can cause you to gain back all the weight you initially lost, and pack on some extra.

It's imperative that you don't fall into this trap of extreme dieting. Does eating nothing make you lose weight? You bet, but in most cases this is only temporary weight loss because you've lost so much muscle by starving yourself. It's more about balance and being smart about your diet, rather than just simply feeding yourself crumbs throughout the day. As I said before, the more muscle you have, the faster your metabolism is going to be. Knowing this, you have to think of muscle as gold. You want to hold onto as much muscle as you possibly can. When trying to lose fat, it's important to have an idea of how many calories you should be expending in a given day. Fat loss is accomplished through calorie deficit (eating less energy than you expend). You can create a calorie deficit either by strictly exercising, strictly dieting, or the best option, which is to do a combination of both.

One pound of fat is equal to roughly 3,500 calories.[15] With this knowledge, and of course eating good healthy foods, weight loss can be broken down into a simple math equation. I've always hated and sucked at math, but this math is simple, I promise you. Knowing that 3,500 calories is roughly equal to one pound of fat, then simple math will tell you that if you have a calorie deficit of 500 calories a day, that will result in a one pound loss by the end of the week. A 1,000 calorie deficit will equal two pounds lost. Determining how many calories you need in a day to at least maintain the weight you are currently at can be done with a simple google search. You will find dozens of options for a calorie calculator.

Generally speaking, a calorie calculator will ask you several questions in order to give you an accurate number of calories that you will need to eat every day to reach specific goals - such as losing weight, maintaining weight, or gaining weight. A calorie calculator will usually ask you for your age, gender, height, your current weight, and activity level. All of these factors go into figuring your daily caloric needs. Activity levels will typically give you different options depending on how often and hard your physical activity is during the week, or whether you are sedentary. As far as activity levels go, don't be a couch potato; you need to get off the couch for the sake of your health, even if you eat flawlessly. It is a good idea to recalculate your caloric needs every week if you have lost or gained any weight.

Another option some calorie calculators will give you is to calculate your basal metabolic rate (BMR). Your basal metabolic rate is basically what your body needs for calories to maintain itself in its current condition when you are just resting. A less scientific term for BMR is simply your resting metabolic rate.[16] As previously said, the more muscle you have, the faster your metabolism will be, this is what affects your basal metabolic rate. Now, when it comes to physical activity, a calorie calculator will give you one of several options you must choose from. Generally speaking, it will give the options of light active (exercise/play sports for one to three times a week), moderately active (exercise/play sports three to five times a week), very active (hard exercise/play sports six to seven times a week), and finally, extra active (you do very hard/intense exercising/play sports, or have a very physical job). The more active you are, the more calories you can consume in a day and still hit your weight loss goals; including losing a safe amount of weight every week until you meet your goals.

For those who don't want to bother doing the math on their own, most calorie calculators will calculate how many calories you need to eat to lose up to two pounds a week, maintain your weight, or to even gain up to two pounds a week. I find calorie calculators very useful and necessary if you are serious about controlling your weight with diet and or exercise. One thing I never recommend is eating below 1,500 calories a day, and never having a calorie deficit of more than 1,000 on any given day. Reducing calories this low, in my opinion, is unnecessary and too extreme. But if you are going borderline extreme with your diet, it's not a bad idea to be taking some vitamin and mineral supplements just to make sure you're getting enough of these essential elements, especially considering you're taking in far less food than normal.[3]

Everyone will have different caloric needs based on the different factors that determine how much an individual requires. However, according to the U.S. Department of Health, the average male adult requires about 2,700 calories a day, and the average adult female requires about 2,200.[17] These calorie markers are a very rough benchmark, and it's interesting to know, but I highly recommend using a calorie calculator to be more precise if you want to get the best results from your diet. On a different note, one thing that I do believe is a waste of time to worry about, or measure, is BMI.

BMI stands for Body Mass Index. The number you see when you measure your BMI is a numerical value of your weight that is in relation to your height.[18] In my opinion, BMI should be banished. It's not a number you ever have to worry about. What BMI doesn't take into consideration is the fact that you can have a lot of muscle, and very little fat. It doesn't break down your body composition to give you an accurate judgment on whether or not you are at a healthy weight for your height. Remember that body composition is the percentages of fat, muscle, bone, and water that your body has. BMI doesn't take any of these factors into consideration. What if you're short, but have a lot of dense, heavy muscle mass? BMI would likely label you as overweight, or even obese! Hell, if you were to measure the BMI of most professional bodybuilders it would tell you that they are obese too! Are you kidding me? Common sense says that someone who has mountains of muscle but so little fat that you can see veins popping out of places most of us just see skin, he/she is without a doubt, not obese. BMI doesn't mean jack.

The numbers that sincerely matter are your composition numbers; your body fat percentage, muscle mass, hydration level, and bone mass (which should stay the same for years, unless you have osteoporosis or some other bone disease). I hate that BMI is still used by professionals today. That unquestionably needs to change. We don't need to be telling people they are obese based on a number that doesn't show the entire picture of what your body is made up of. Now, with that being said, I do recommend other measurements you should be doing once a week to properly track the effects of your dieting and workout programs.

Measuring certain body parts on a regular basis will help you see if your body is changing or not - and if that change is in the direction you want it to be headed in. Other measurements to take notice of, besides your weight and body fat, are the changes in the size of your arms, thighs, waist, and hips. You may need the help of a second hand to do these measurements. You can certainly try to do them on your own, but that may be a bit challenging.

Here's how you should measure each of the major body parts mentioned above:

To measure the arms, take a tape measure and simply wrap it around the center of both your biceps and triceps on each arm.[112]

Measuring your thighs consists of taking the tape measure and wrapping it around the middle of your thighs (midway between your knees and hip).[112]

To measure your waist, run the tape measure just above your belly button but below your ribcage.[112]

 Finally, to measure your hips, you need to take the tape measure and run it around the fullest part of your hips and butt.[112]

I would recommend doing these measurements along with measuring your weight and body fat once a week.

All of the things I have mentioned in this chapter (measuring body fat, your arms, waist, hips, thighs, and paying the most attention to noticeable changes in the mirror), are all much more important than obsessing over the scale. The scale is the least important thing on this list of things you should be measuring and paying attention to every week. Yes, use it, but the scale is the device that tells you the least and can make you unnecessarily worry the most.

Chapter Four Summary:

- **Don't obsess over your weight or step on that scary scale every day. It's not healthy for you psychologically.**

- **Your weight can fluctuate within a few pounds every day because of three main factors: water retention, bodily waste** accumulation, and the food you have eaten throughout the day.

- Weighing yourself every day can cause panic to set in, especially if you happen to weigh yourself during a weight fluctuation, due to the factors mentioned above. The above factors are why it's not recommended to weigh yourself daily.

- It's better to pay attention to changes in the mirror than a number on a scale. Be patient; changes are slow and subtle, but well worth the wait when you see them.

- Instead of daily weigh-ins, weigh yourself no more than once a week, and look for the trend over time. Is your weight going down, up, or staying relatively the same? Don't be alarmed if you don't hit your goals every week due to natural weight fluctuation.

- Using a body-fat analyzer along with a weight scale is the best way to go since fat loss, rather than just strictly body weight loss, should be your true goal when trying to lose weight. You can buy body-fat analyzer online for a reasonable price, and some weight scales have one built right into them.

- The best time to weigh yourself is first thing in the morning, after you have gone to the bathroom, with little to no clothing, and before you have eaten anything. This will give you the most accurate body weight measurement. The worst time to weigh yourself is at night.

- The sweet spot of weight loss for the best long-term results are to lose one to two pounds of fat per week. Anything more may be too fast.

- Losing too much weight too fast likely means you are using too much muscle for energy rather than mostly fat. This is detrimental, considering that the amount of muscle you have is directly linked to the speed of your metabolism.

- It can take up to six weeks to start seeing results when first starting a new diet or exercise regimen. This is due to the fact that you are putting a sudden stress on your body, and it can react by holding onto water to protect muscle tissue. If you do not start seeing results after six weeks of exercising or dieting, check with your doctor for a possible underlying medical condition.

- It may be wise to check with your doctor if it seems impossible to not only lose weight but to gain weight as well. This may be a sign of the thyroid gland not behaving normally.

- It is not uncommon to lose much more than the recommended one to two pounds a week when you first start dieting and exercising. This is likely due to your body disposing of water retention. After the first few weeks, your weight loss numbers should normalize. It's important to know this, so you are not overexcited in the beginning and then disappointed when things normalize.

- Don't be overly strict with your diet. This is the number one way to incidentally burn up badly needed muscle for energy, rather than fat, because your body will go into "starvation mode".

- Commonly, what happens when people borderline starve themselves is yes, they do lose weight, but when they begin to eat normally again, they will usually gain it all back and pack on extra weight. The reasoning behind this is because their bodies now have a slower metabolism because their bodies have eaten up some muscle for energy.

- 3,500 calories equals approximately one pound of fat. This means that if you diet and/or exercise enough and you have a

500 calorie deficit every day, you will lose one pound a week. A 1,000 calorie deficit a day will net you a loss of two pounds a week.

- A calorie calculator is a useful tool to determine your caloric needs accurately. They will also normally do the math for you if you are looking to lose, or even gain, up to two pounds a week. Recalculate your caloric needs every week if you have lost or gained any weight. A good calorie calculator can be found with a simple google search online.

- I never recommend eating below 1,500 calories per day, or a calorie deficit of more than 1,000 a day either. Reducing calorie intake to this low is too extreme in my opinion.

- If you are going borderline extreme with your diet and/or exercising, I recommend taking vitamin and mineral supplements just to make sure you are getting enough of these essential elements.

- Ignore your BMI (Body Mass Index), which is a numeric value of your weight in relation to your height, and know this; according to BMI, bodybuilders are obese.

- Rather than paying attention to useless BMI numbers, the important numbers to watch out for are your body composition factors: body fat percentage, muscle mass, water/hydration levels, and bone mass.

- On top of your weekly weigh-ins and measuring body fat, doing weekly measurements of your arms, thighs, waist, and hips will help you track the results of your dieting and/or workout programs.

- Out of all the things to measure and pay attention to, the mirror is the most important, and the scale is the least important.

Chapter Five: *The Workout/Diet Connection – Hint: Their Dating*

Lesson 5: Thinking you can eat whatever you want as long as you work out is a zero sum game.

It wasn't until I was in my 30's when it seemed as though I was no longer burning food off as fast as it hit my mouth. It was during this time that I came to the realization that even though I busted my ass working out, I could no longer continue to eat whatever I wanted and still get impressive results in the gym. This was around the same time that I decided to take my passion for health and fitness and try to turn it into a living. So, I earned my personal training certification, which I still hold to this day. When I hit my 30's it seemed as though my body was going through a "slow down" as my age started creeping away from my physical prime years. At this time I truly began to research the effect of diet on the body. I especially studied the effect of my diet on my workouts, since they were no longer as effective with the same careless eating I had in my testosterone fueled teens and twenties. That and my personal training certification course included formal education on diet along with the physical exercise/activity training. These proved to be both interesting and extremely eye opening.

This mistake of thinking that you can eat whatever you want as long as you work out may not have a noticeable effect in your younger years, but the human body does slow down over time no matter how well you treat it. Tom Brady of the Patriots football team, may seem to be someone who could still throw a football well into his 40's, will eventually slow down physically. He is infamous for dieting in such a way as to keep himself at the top of his game for as long as possible. He has been tremendously effective at this with the help of a fantastic personal chef.

We may not all be able to afford a personal chef, but with focus and determination anyone can choose to eat the right healthy foods. Also, even though you may experience what I have, which is to eat less than stellar during your younger years and still look great and get impressive results from working out, there will come a point in time when that will change. I can promise you that. Not only that, but the better you eat, the better you can work out, and the results you can achieve will be even greater. Remember this fact before thinking of shoveling down whatever food you want if you work out; roughly 80 percent of what your physique looks like is directly related to the foods you eat, and 20 percent is linked to daily physical activity and exercise.[19] This 80-20 rule is a physiological fact that points to how important food is if you want to stick out at the beach.

I often wish I wouldn't have had the mentality of thinking I could eat anything I wanted to and still look my best when I was in my prime. I have been able to get amazing results with my efforts in the gym even without a great diet in the past, but my results could have potentially been even better if I had not been so naïve on the subject of food. However, I learned from my mistakes, and that is in part the motivation for writing this book;

to teach others about the errors that I have made so that they can be avoided.

Chapter Five Summary:

- **Just because you work out, it doesn't mean you get a free pass to eat whatever you want.**

- **During your younger years, you may not notice the effect of eating too much junk, but your body will "slow down, " and it will become more apparent in your older years with either weight gain, health problems, or both. Your 30's are when you start aging away from your prime, but even in your younger years, it's important to eat right for health and optimal body composition (fat, muscle, bone, and water percentages).**

- **The better you eat, the better you can look and feel. Also, you can attain better results from working out.**

- **80 percent of what your physique looks like is directly related to your diet; the other 20 percent is linked to physical activity and exercise.**

Chapter Six: *Delicious Regret*

Lesson 6: Sugar, the eighth deadly sin.

Out of all the things you can eat, refined added sugar is one of, if not the, worst thing you can ever put into your body.[20] Eating too many added sugars is perhaps the most disastrous diet blunder you can make and it will kill your chances of having any real success with your diet. Added sugars are essentially calories with no nutrients, or "empty calories," and they can hurt your metabolism in the long run.[20] Added sugars are non-naturally occurring sugars that food manufacturers add for flavor. Regular table sugar, also known as sucrose, is a good example of an added sugar you can put in or on foods yourself. Another common added sugar is high fructose corn syrup. Sugars that occur naturally in things like fruits or milk are fine to eat because they are natural, unrefined, and they come with many nutrients. The fiber in things like fruits slows the effect of sugar on blood sugar levels.[21]

Sugar in moderation is somewhat manageable, but moderation and sugar rarely go hand in hand. Sweets and sugar are a slow killer. Just eating one candy bar is probably not going to have any immediate or long lasting effect on your body, but eating too much junk over time can certainly lead to disease and obesity. Part of the problem with sugar and unhealthy foods is that it doesn't make you sick or fat as soon as it touches your lips. If it did, you would see a lot less food related health problems. Just imagine if having one bowl of ice cream gave you an instant heart attack. Ice cream would be no more. Since it doesn't work like that, and disease from poor diet happens slowly over time, this compounds the obesity crisis that's become so widespread in this country.

Sugar has such a strong addictive hold on so many people. Believe it or not, sugar is considered more addicting than cocaine.[22] It even stimulates the same area of the brain that addictive drugs do.[23] This powerful addictive nature of sugar is likely the reason why sugar cravings can be incredibly intense and so difficult to overcome. Sugar cravings are a real addiction and a real problem, especially in America. I know this all too well first hand. I've struggled with sugar addiction since I was a kid. I've had moments in life where it seemed I'd beaten sugar, but indulging my sweet tooth before completely being able to retrain my taste buds has always resulted in a relapse. It takes quite a force of willpower to subdue a sugar addiction.

The only way to truly beat an addiction is to avoid it altogether. That's what makes addictions so hard to overcome. It's the same as being a smoker; unless you completely refrain from touching cigarettes, it will be nearly impossible to quit! Sugar is no different than any other kind of addiction; avoidance is the only path to victory, or at least weeding it out of your diet long enough so that you can avoid it and not relapse with intense cravings. Now, the amount of sugar that is consumed in a typical diet here in the U.S. is astounding.

People are consuming an average of over 60 pounds of added sugar a year, with a typical daily intake of over 70 grams of added sugar a day, which is more than twice the recommended limit![24] That right there is an enormous amount of added sugar. This mass consumption of sugar is a huge cause of the obesity epidemic in our society today. Excessive sugar consumption can lead to all kinds of problems that are related to obesity, such as type II diabetes, cardiovascular disease, and many other diseases.[24] Eating far too many added sugars is a huge reason so many people in this country are overweight and sick. According to the American Heart Association the maximum amount of added sugar you should eat in a day for men is 150 calories (38 grams, or nine teaspoons), 100 calories for women (25 grams a day, or six teaspoons), and only three to six teaspoons of sugar for kids (20 to 25 grams).[25] Children's upper sugar limits depend on their age and how many calories they need.[25] When you think of it in terms of small teaspoons of sugar, that is not a lot of sugar you should eat in a day.

If it were up to me, I would say the daily recommended amount of added sugar would be zero grams. Added sugars in our lovely American food makes this nearly impossible unless you can afford to buy only whole natural foods which, let's be honest, can run the grocery bill up pretty high. That's the best way to eat, but not always affordable for low-income families. As hard as it may be, it is ideal if you can do everything in your power to avoid foods that have added sugar, especially if you want to lose weight and optimize your health. It is important to point out that although the American Heart Association says you can safely consume a certain amount of added sugar, your body has zero need for them to be in your diet as they serve no physiological purpose.[26] The less you eat, the better you will feel and the healthier you will be. On top of all that, you have to watch out for foods that are labeled "healthy," "natural," or low fat.

Frequently, what happens with so-called "healthy" foods are the exact opposite of what a real healthy option would be. These foods, and low-fat or diet foods, have often had fat removed from them. To replace the lost flavor sugar and other junk ingredients must be added to make it so the food doesn't taste like total crap.[25] Fat is not the devil. Fat needs to be a part of your diet in the right quantities, and there are healthy fats in things like fish and nuts that have essential nutrients that your body needs.[27] Just eating fat isn't going to make you fat unless you consume too much, but undoubtedly too much of anything is bad. Saturated fat is the worst kind of fat though, so it's good to limit this as it is considered the artery clogging kind of fat.[27] However, sugar is worse for you than fat.[24] Sugar = enemy number one. You can find added sugar in all sorts of foods that are commonly viewed as healthy, such as yogurt, bread, etc. Sugar isn't always known as "sugar" though. Sugar has many names, some of which you may have never heard of.

When looking at ingredients, there are at least an astounding 61 names for sugar you need to watch out for.[28] In fact, over 70 percent of packaged foods contain added sugars.[28] Besides the common names of sugar I've already mentioned, things like barley malt, dextrose, maltose, and a whole slew of other names are given for sugar. For a complete list of the 61 names of sugar to watch out for visit this website:[28] http://sugarscience.ucsf.edu/hidden-in-plain-sight/#.W_c-NDhKjIU

An excellent way to cut back on sugar is to do everything you can to avoid processed foods, and if you're craving something sweet then reach for some fruit. If you do reach for fruit make sure you choose fresh fruits instead of fruits that are canned in syrup, which is just unneeded and added sugar. Also, avoid these so called healthy sugars: agave, organic cane sugar, and coconut sugar. Don't be tricked into thinking these are healthy. They are still plain old sugar without the nutrients you get from other foods with sugar such as fruits. However, some natural sweeteners are perfectly fine for you to eat.

An excellent example of a natural zero-calorie alternative to sugar is stevia. Other alternatives to sugar are things like cinnamon, nutmeg, almond extract, vanilla, ginger, or lemon. One last thing I'd like to mention is a word about sugar alcohols. These don't actually have anything to do with alcohol, so they won't get you drunk, but they are a better option for you than regular refined sugar.[29] Let me explain how. First, there are several different types of sugar alcohols, but the most popular ones are xylitol, erythritol, sorbitol, and maltitol.[29]

Sugar alcohols are a replacement for sugar. They can be found naturally occurring in some fruits and vegetables, but most sugar alcohols are less sweet than regular refined sugar, and they metabolize much slower too.[30] They are a hybrid of sugar and alcohol, but you won't find these at the bar.[29] Sugar alcohols have fewer calories than regular sugar and they have other benefits as well.[29] Sugar alcohols don't raise your blood sugar nearly as much as regular sugar does.[29] This is good news for people with diabetes. They are better for your teeth as well.[29] As we all know, regular sugar can lead to fantastic tooth decay.

However, just because sugar alcohols have some benefits to them, this does not mean you can just go ahead and mow down on them. Consume them in reasonable quantities just as you would anything else. You especially don't want to go too excessive with sugar alcohols as they have been known to cause digestive problems when eaten in high quantities.[29] Each person will have different sensitivity levels to sugar alcohols, but generally speaking, you do not want to eat more than 50 grams in a day; and not more than 30 grams in one sitting.[31] If you want to avoid multiple trips to the bathroom, use sugar alcohols lightly.

When done in moderation, replacing regular sugar with sugar alcohols is a smart choice. Also, I would like to reiterate that limiting or simply eliminating added sugars from your diet can have a tremendously positive effect on your health and weight. Sugar is such a huge problem in this country. I sincerely believe this country would be far healthier if we would stop stripping food of all fat just to replace it with sugar and other ingredients. To recap, remember that if you crave something sweet, reach for some fresh fruit, and give yourself some time to retrain your brain and taste buds to enjoy other foods.

As I've stated before, it is quite okay to eat plenty of foods like fruits and vegetables even though they have sugar and carbs. Our country is going through a phase of carb-phobia. You need carbs in your diet; they are not the enemy, junk carbs from crap food is. However, not all carbs are created equal. Yes, avoid bad carbs from junk and sweets, but you don't ever need to cut fruits and vegetables right out of your diet. I'm strongly against any diet that suggests doing this for long-term. Certain diets do suggest going very low on carbs for a small amount of time to trick your body into burning fat. These are a rare exception because there is a legitimate science to these kinds of diets,[32] but if a diet says you need to cut out fruits and veggies for an extended period of time, throw that diet plan right in the garbage.

Finally, fight the urge to give into temptation while trying to curb a sugar addiction. That cupcake may sound like some kind of deliciousness, but think of it this way, what are you going to have to do to burn that off if you're trying to be healthy and lose weight? Take the time to think to yourself, how many stair climbers am I going to have to do to burn that cupcake off? How many miles am I going to have to run to burn that cake, ice cream, soda, or what have you, off. If you make it a habit of thinking like this before you consider scarfing down any tasty foods, I think you will find your willpower will ratchet up a notch. Lastly, if you find yourself struggling with food cravings, remember this quip; sweets and junk food are just fleeting moments of pleasure, which will often later turn into delicious regret.

Chapter Six Summary:

- **Refined added sugar is perhaps the worst thing you can put into your body. It's calories with no nutrients, and too much of them can hurt your metabolism over time.**

- **Eating too many added sugars is perhaps the worst diet blunder you can make.**

- **Naturally occurring sugars in things like fruit and milk are fine to eat. They are natural, unrefined, and they come with nutrients and fiber.**

- Sugar in moderation is manageable, but too many sweets and sugar in your diet are a slow killer.

- Sugar is considered more addictive than cocaine. It stimulates the same area of the brain that addictive drugs do.

- Sugar addiction is a real problem. The only way to truly beat an addiction is to get to the point where you can completely avoid it altogether.

- The average consumption of sugar in the U.S. is over 60 pounds per person every year. Too much added sugar can make you fat and sick. Deadly diseases such as type II diabetes, cardiovascular disease, and many others can be attributed to a high sugar diet.

- Although it is difficult to afford wholesome and healthy foods if you're on a budget, you should still do everything in your power to avoid food with added sugars in it. This can assist you to lose weight and optimize health.

- Although the American Heart Association states you can safely have some added sugars in your diet, your body has no need for added sugars. They don't serve any physiological purpose.

- Watch out for foods that are labeled "healthy", "natural", or low fat. Often these foods are stripped of flavorful fat and replaced with sugar and other junk ingredients to enhance flavor that is actually worse for you than the fat food manufacturers strip from foods.

- Some fat IS needed in your diet. Healthy fats are in things like nuts and fish that come with nutrients. Limit saturated fat though; this is the artery clogging kind of fat.

- Sugar is worse for you than fat. You can find added sugars in foods typically thought of as healthy such as yogurt, bread, and many others.

- There are over 61 names for sugar that you can find in the ingredients on nutritional labels. Some of the most common names for sugar are sucrose, high fructose corn syrup, dextrose, and many others. You can find a full list of the names for sugar by visiting this website: http://sugarscience.ucsf.edu/hidden-in-plain-sight/#.W_c-NDhKjIU

- You can find added sugar in over 70 percent of packaged food.

- One of the best ways to avoid added sugar is to cut back on processed food. If you crave something sweet, reach for some fresh fruit, but not fruit that's canned in syrup.

- Avoid so-called "healthy" sugars such as agave, organic cane sugar, and coconut sugar. These are not healthy for you.

- Some natural sweeteners are a good alternative to sugar. Stevia is a good one with zero calories. Other alternatives are things like cinnamon, nutmeg, almond extract, vanilla, ginger (which is good for your stomach, think back to when you were sick), honey, or lemon.

- Sugar alcohols are a good replacement for sugar; they won't make you drunk though. They are found occurring naturally in some fruits and veggies, but most sugar alcohols are less sweet than regular refined sugar.

- Sugar alcohols are a hybrid of sugar and alcohol, have fewer calories and won't raise your blood sugar levels nearly as much as regular sugar. This alternative to regular sugar is suitable for people with diabetes and they're better for your teeth as well.

- Although sugar alcohols contain fewer calories and have other benefits to regular sugar, go easy on them. They can cause digestive issues when consumed in high quantities.

- Everyone will have different sensitivity levels to sugar alcohols, but try not to eat more than 50 grams a day, or 30 grams in one sitting, as this may prompt multiple trips to the bathroom.

- To recap, reach for some fresh fruit and give your brain and taste buds time to retrain themselves to enjoy other non-sugary foods.

- Don't fall for carb-phobia. You need carbs. Not all carbs are created equal. Avoid junk carbs from crap food, but carbs from good foods like fruits and vegetables are a must. Some diets recommend very low carbs at the beginning of the diet plan. This is fine, as there is a real science to this, but it's only temporary. Never do a diet that cuts fruits and vegetables out of your diet for a prolonged period of time.

- **Fight the urge to give into temptation if you're battling a sugar addiction. Think of it in terms of what needs to be done to burn junk food or sweets if you are trying to be healthy and lose weight. How many miles are you going to have to run to burn off that cake? Think of it in these terms before indulging.**

- **Sweets and junk food are just fleeting moments of pleasure, which often later turn into delicious regret.**

Chapter Seven: *Supper Timing*

Lesson 7: Do not eat at least three hours before bedtime.

Eating late at night has been one of the hardest mistakes I've personally had to overcome, and to be honest, I still struggle with this kitchen blunder from time to time. The times when I have been the most successful in not eating too close to bedtime have been the times when I have had the most success with my diet. It has never been easy though, far from it. I always find that I am hungrier at night. I have an astounding ability to be great with my diet all day, but as soon as things start to wind down at night, or if I get bored, hunger sets in. For me, hunger from boredom or lack of activity happens at night more than any other times during the day.

There are only a couple of ways that I have found that work in overcoming the late night eating/snacking struggle. One is to either do the best you can to keep yourself distracted from thinking about food. The other way of beating the late night eating difficulties comes down to just practicing sheer force of willpower to not eat at night when you know you're not supposed to. Staying busy can help you be distracted from the feeling of hunger; especially when it comes to what's called emotional eating, or comfort food.[33] Just plopping down in front of the couch is probably the worst thing you can do. It's the easiest thing to do, and I admit I've been guilty of this more times than I can count, but you need to try to stay busy up until an hour or so before bedtime. At least an hour or so of not being busy will give you some down time, so you're not too stimulated when you try to get some shuteye. Some of us fortunate ones don't have this problem of being hungrier at night. As for me, I seem to be a night owl naturally, so it's been a challenge that's popped its ugly head up a lot in the past. Eating too close to bed is a problem for a couple of different reasons.

If you eat too close to bedtime, the food you eat is more than likely going to be stored as fat that you have to work off later if you want to get that perfect beach physique.[3] Another reason why you don't want to eat too close to bed is that it can mess with your sleep, and don't underestimate the importance of sleep. You need those ideal eight hours of sleep at night. Sleep is crucial for hormone regulation and your metabolism.[34] Numerous workings in your body don't function right when you are sleep deprived.[34] Your health, energy levels, weight, and mood can all be adversely affected by too little sleep.[34] Since eating too close to bedtime can disturb your sleep, let's go over what can go wrong with your body when you operate on a lack of sleep.

One thing that can get out of whack if you are sleep deprived is that it can alter what's called your glucose tolerance.[34] In the interest of not getting too scientific, I'll explain this in simple terms. First, glucose is sugar that carbohydrates are broken down into which ends up floating around in your bloodstream.[35] Glucose tolerance is basically how readily your body's cells can recognize glucose in your bloodstream, pull it into the cells throughout your body, and then use that as needed fuel for the cells of your body to operate correctly.[3] What happens with too little sleep is that that your glucose tolerance becomes impaired.[34] Glucose intolerance is a nasty side effect of sleep deprivation that can leave you feeling tired and hungry, which can make you want to reach for food more often, creating a calorie surplus, which of course leads to weight gain.[36] This is all happening because your body's cells are not operating at peak efficiency due to the fact that your glucose tolerance is out of whack. Hormone regulation is affected by lack of sleep as well.

Sleep deprivation can lead to your body lowering the hormone *leptin* and increase the hormone *ghrelin*.[34] Leptin is an appetite-suppressing hormone that your fat cells produce, and this hormone is usually produced the most at night.[34] Ghrelin is a hormone that your stomach releases that stimulates the feeling of hunger.[34] To make matters worse, while your appetite is acting something fierce due to lack of sleep, your body is going to want quick energy to feel alive and wake up. For this reason, you are more likely to crave sweets when you haven't slept well.[37] A lack of sleep can also throw your cortisol hormone levels off as well.[34] Cortisol levels that are too high have been shown to increase belly fat and can lead to other health problems such as diabetes.[38]

As you can see, sufficient sleep is vital, and since eating too close to bed can not only lead to fat accumulation as well as sleep deprivation (and all the lovely side effects that come with that), make sure you do your very best to get a good, quality eight hours of sleep every night. Challenging in today's world? Yes, but unfortunately our bodies still require the same amount of sleep as they always have. I wish that could change and we could evolve to live and operate our best on little to no sleep. Imagine how much we could get done. Alas, that's not going to happen, so let's not fight a battle we can't win. However, I do believe we can wage a winnable war on obesity, diabetes, heart disease, and all of the negative consequences that can result from a poor diet. Not eating at least three hours before bedtime is another battle that you must win. Eating too late at night is an obstacle among many other obstacles you must learn to overcome if you want to achieve whatever goals are pertaining to your diet you may have.

Chapter Seven Summary:

- **Avoid eating at least three hours before bedtime.**

- **Staying busy can help you be distracted from late night hunger, or simply sheer force of willpower can prevent you from indulging.**

- **Food that is consumed too close to bedtime will likely be stored as body fat.**

- **Eating too close to bedtime can cause sleep disturbance. Sleep deprivation can lead to a host of problems you need to avoid if you want diet success.**

- Sleep is important for your health, weight, energy levels, mood, hormone regulation, and metabolism efficiency. All of which can have an effect on how easy it is to regulate your diet, and how your body performs on a daily basis.

- Lack of sleep can wreak havoc on certain inner workings of your body. Glucose tolerance and hormone regulation can be affected by being deprived of sleep.

- Glucose tolerance impairment can result from lack of sleep. This can lead to tiredness and more feelings of hunger than normal because your body's cells are not operating correctly. Your body will crave sweets more when you are tired. If you indulge these cravings, this can have an adverse effect on your health and weight.

- With a lack of sleep, the hormone Leptin, an appetite-suppressing hormone, will decrease. Ghrelin, an appetite-increasing hormone, will rise along with cortisol, a hormone, when produced in excess, is known to increase belly fat and other health problems.

Chapter Eight: *The Waterboy Was a Genius*

Lesson 8: Stay hydrated. I repeat, stay hydrated.

It just can't be said enough; you need to stay hydrated. Virtually every chemical reaction that takes place in your body requires water to function properly.[39] If you are dehydrated, it's impossible for your body and metabolism to perform at peak levels.[3] In fact, mental performance and physical coordination can start to become impaired if you lose just one percent of your body's water![40] This starts to occur before you even begin to feel thirsty, which happens when you have lost about two to three percent of your body's water.[3] The human body is made up of anywhere from 60 to 75 percent water.[41] That number can vary based on things like age, gender, how much fat you carry, or how lean you are.[42]

Dehydration can lead to a host of problems or bothersome symptoms. For starters, being dehydrated can make you feel sluggish and tired throughout the day.[43] On the other hand, if you keep yourself fully hydrated and eat properly, chances are you are going to be feeling much better than if you aren't drinking enough fluids; the right fluids I might add. Also, your digestive system will operate much better if you are fully hydrated.[44] There are so many benefits to drinking plenty of water that it's hard to count them.

Research has shown that if you were to drink just water for fluids for nine days straight, you could lose weight faster.[45] You could end up losing the same amount of calories than if you jogged for over half a mile every day for those nine days because you aren't taking in any extra calories from fluids. Also, drinking plenty of water can help you concentrate better. The human brain is made up of about 75 to 85 percent water, so drinking water helps to fuel and maintain it.[45] Drinking water can also contribute to suppressing your appetite by filling your belly, which can lead to weight loss.[45] Your body will flush out toxins faster if you drink lots of water as well.[45] Washing out these harmful substances with water can slow down the aging process.[45]

Water can also help lower the risk of many diseases, hypertension (high blood pressure), bladder conditions, and bowel cancer, to name a few.[45] Water can also help your heart work better. Just five glasses of water a day has shown to reduce the risk of a heart attack by up to 41 percent.[45] Finally, your skin becomes softer and cleaner because water can help to clear and moisten the skin.[45] These are just some of the many benefits of our most critical fluid, water. One thing to remember about drinking water is never to reuse plastic water bottles you buy from the store. These are meant for a one-time use only. The plastic material can leach into the water if you reuse it and this is known to increase the chances of developing cancer.[46] Rather than reuse plastic bottles, you can buy reusable bottles for relatively cheap, but make sure you buy one that is BPA free. So, how much water should you be drinking in a day?

Unfortunately, everyone's body is different, so the amount of water you need to be drinking is entirely dependent on your specific needs based on a few different criteria. The standard eight, eight ounce glasses of water a day simply does not suffice. Since no two bodies are exactly identical, your hydration needs are naturally going to be different. The old cliché of eight glasses a day may be sufficient for some people, but for others, it's simply not enough. Your H2O needs are dependent on three different things.

Your weight, activity level, and climate all have a direct impact on how much fluids you should be drinking every day.[3] Keep in mind that all three of these variables can change. Typically, if you take your weight and divide it in half, that's how many ounces of water you should be drinking in a day.[3] This is a good general rule of thumb, but don't ignore the other two factors for your hydration needs as well. With this rule of half your body weight in ounces, for someone who weighs 200 pounds, their basic hydration need should be at the very minimum 100 ounces of water a day. If you were to go by the standard eight glasses, eight ounces each, a day, you would fall short by at least 36 ounces. That's a lot of water your body needs that it's not getting. And this is just your base number;

the other factors, activity level, and climate can make that amount of ounces go up closer to an ounce of water needed for every pound of body weight.

Naturally, the more active you are, the more water your body is going to need. If you are sweating like crazy because you play physically intense sports, or you're working out at a very extreme level, you will need to up your fluid intake. The climate you live or work in matters too. If you live in a hot climate, you should be drinking more water, especially if you a very active. If you live in a colder climate, you probably won't need as much water. Although, a dry climate, whether hot or cold, will make your hydration needs go up as well. Keep in mind that in really cold and dry climates, every time you are outside breathing in that cold, dry air, water leaves your body on every exhale.[3] Because of these reasons, you need to make extra sure you are drinking plenty of water. Now, there are plenty of do's and don'ts when it comes to hydration.

One thing that I recommend is to drink an entire glass of cold water immediately after you wake up in the morning. Research has shown that by drinking a full glass of cold water first thing in the morning is for one, a good way to wake yourself up, and it's also shown to give your metabolism a sudden, small, temporary boost.[47] It's not going to give you enough of a boost that you'll shed some serious pounds, but it certainly doesn't hurt either. Notice how I said cold water too, not warm. Drinking cold water is another thing you can do to give your metabolism a slight temporary boost.

Anytime you drink or eat anything that is different than your body's temperature, your body has to work a little bit to get whatever it is you ate or drank to match the internal temperature of your body.[48] Your body has to use some energy to heat up cold water. However, this is trivial, since it does not take very long or a ton of energy to warm up some cold water once you have drank it, but every little tip or trick can help if you are trying to lose weight or look your best. I also want to point out that muscle contains more water than fat, which means the leaner you are, the higher your water needs are going to be.[3] It's also interesting to point out that sometimes when you feel hungry, it may actually be a sign of thirst.

The same area of the brain that controls hunger also controls thirst, so it's easy to get the two confused.[49] Unless there's an obvious reason you would feel hungry, such as not eating all day, it's not a terrible idea to first drink a glass of water when you're feeling hungry. Wait a few minutes after drinking to see if your hunger subsides. If your hunger does subside then chances are thirst was the real culprit. By doing this, you can prevent unnecessarily eating extra calories when your body isn't truly telling you it's time to eat. Also, being fully hydrated at all times in the first place can help prevent this brain hunger/thirst confusion. Now when it comes to drinking anything other than water, there are some important things to remember.

One thing that I don't recommend you drink in most circumstances is Gatorade. Now, why wouldn't Gatorade be something that would be considered ok to drink? After all, athletes are well known to drink this stuff right? Yes, that is true. I remember the old Gatorade commercials. While Gatorade certainly does have essential electrolytes in it, it also has sugar that you simply do not need. You can make an electrolyte drink right from plain old home ingredients; you don't need to go out and buy Gatorade.[3]

The added sugar is the only reason why I don't recommend drinking Gatorade. Of course, there is an exception. Athletes do drink this stuff for a reason, especially professional athletes. Athletes perform at extremely high levels, and they sometimes sweat like crazy. If you are doing work or exercising to the point you are dripping in sweat, reaching for a Gatorade is not a horrible idea; if you haven't made your own homemade electrolyte concoction that is. Sweating makes you lose electrolytes, but if you are not seriously sweating your ass off, there is no need to drink the unneeded sugar you will get with the Gatorade.[50] Another thing you certainly don't need is soda.

Soda is plain horrible for you. You probably knew that, but it's worth mentioning. For one, they are loaded with sugar. You could pretty much call soda liquid sugar with some additives. Have you ever looked at the nutritional label of a Mountain Dew? Just one 20 ounce bottle is a whopping 77 grams of sugar! That's about 15 teaspoons of sugar. That's insane! That is far more grams of sugar than is recommended in a day, and the highest amount of any sodas last time I checked. I use to love this stuff. When I was younger, I use to drink this stuff quite frequently. Now, I rarely drink any soda at all, and it's one of the first things I recommend people cut out when trying to diet the right way. You don't need that awfulness in your life. And it's not just the sugar in soda that's bad; there's a ton of caffeine in them as well. If you value sleep, especially if you're sensitive to caffeine like I am, I'd surely steer clear of soda. Just a small amount of caffeine gives me the shakes, and I get anxious as hell. Needless to say, I rarely drink any soda or coffee, another fluid I will touch on later.

I don't even recommend drinking ginger ale when you are sick. Remember when you were a kid and your parents use to tell you to drink ginger ale if you got the flu or any other kind of bug? Well, that was not the best piece of advice our parents had for us. Ginger ale, like any soda, has sugar in it, so you should be avoiding it. If you are sick, the best fluid to be taking is straight up water.[51] Although there are ginger ale brands that claim they have real ginger in them. Ginger does have health benefits, including soothing an upset stomach.[52] However, you do not need to drink ginger ale to get some ginger in your system. Now, another bad thing about soda are those pesky things called calories. Don't you hate those little devils?

It's amazing how many and how quickly you can consume calories just from drinking things like soda, fruit juice, coffee loaded with crème and sugar, or basically anything but pure water. Often the amount of calories that one consumes in fluid form are drastically overlooked or underestimated. However, being calorie conscious does not mean you should reach for a diet soda instead of regular soda.

Diet soda may be worse for you than the regular soda with plain old sugar in it. The crap they put in diet soda, like aspartame, is terrible for you; I'd never recommend drinking it.[53] Another negative about caffeinated soda is that it is a diuretic, which means that even though it does contain water, it can lead you to pee more than if you just drank plain water .[54]

With all this being said, of course, the best course of action is to completely avoid putting any soda into your system at all. I do realize that if you're a soda-aholic, this is not an easy thing to just up and quit. In cases like this, it may be far more feasible to weed soda out of your life slowly until you can come to the point of avoiding it altogether. Instead of drinking eight cokes a day, reduce that number by one every other day and eventually you'll get to the point where you can quit that junk without having extreme cravings. Now, one thing that people have a different opinion about is drinking coffee, which is one of the most consumed beverages in the world.

I'm not personally a coffee drinker, but I do advocate for its benefits, but oppose the added sugars and creamers too often found in coffee drinks. A lot of people assume that coffee is not good for you, but this is a big misconception. What gives coffee its bad name isn't the coffee itself, but all those spoonfuls after spoonfuls of sugar and cream. Coffee in moderation does have a few significant benefits. For starters, it does exactly what most people drink it for; it wakes you the hell up. It gives you a temporary metabolic boost by jolting you with caffeine, which is known to be a stimulant.[55] This benefit is temporary of course, but it isn't a bad thing as long as you don't drink it by the gallon or have an IV hooked up to you pumping you full of coffee. Research also suggests that coffee drinkers benefit from memory enhancement and better mental acuity from their morning cup of joe.[56] Now, the best way to drink coffee is straight up black. To some, this might sound awful, and it kind of is, but you still get all the benefits of coffee without the added crap calories of cream and sugar, and sugar and cream, and cream, and sugar, you get the point.

Unfortunately, too much of anything is a bad thing, even if it's considered healthy; coffee certainly being no exception.

Too much of this popular stimulant (coffee) and you might be paying for it at bedtime, as we all know. Also, coffee is a diuretic just like soda. Coffee and soda are not the only beverages that are diuretics, or beverages that should be limited, though. Alcohol is another diuretic that, if consumed enough, can make you dehydrated.[57] It can also make you feel like crap, especially that wonderful hangover that most of us have certainly experienced once or many times in our lives. It is without a doubt ok to let loose now and again, but drinking too frequently can put you in a state of perpetual dehydration. This is horrible for your health and of course can lead to liver problems, as well as a host of other health problems. So it goes without saying that you should limit alcohol. Except on special occasions, I don't recommend going above the standard recommendation of one drink a day for women and men over the age of 65, and two for men 65 and younger.[57] Alcohol in moderation does have some benefits, especially red wine, which is considered good for your heart if you drink it occasionally. Another beverage that you should limit, or not drink at all, is fruit juice.

Many consider fruit juice a healthy choice. While it is not the worst beverage choice you can make, it's not a wise choice either. This might sound bizarre to some, but there are good reasons that I don't recommend you drink fruit juice, especially if you are trying to lose weight. The problem with fruit juice is that it is mostly sugar. It does have more nutritional value than something like soda, but it is loaded with sugar without the fiber that comes with eating a whole piece of fruit.[3]

A glass of fruit juice has more sugar in it than just one piece of its equivalent fruit. For example, a glass of apple juice has much more sugar in it because the juice comes from several apples, not just one. It is much better for you and your blood sugar levels to eat the whole piece of fruit than drink the fruit juice because, even though it still has sugar in it, the fiber that comes with whole fruits will help to slow down the absorption of the sugar.[58] I will also point out that the sugar that you find in fruits isn't the same as something like refined table sugar. Fruit contains natural sugar, not the refined crap you put in coffee, cereal, or things of that nature. However, a glass of something like apple juice has many more calories and contains no fiber, as opposed to if you simply ate one apple. Stick with eating your fruits, not drinking them. I will add that another benefit of eating fruit is that they usually have a good amount of water in them.

If you are eating the right way, and especially if you eat plenty of fruits and veggies, about 20 percent of your fluid needs should come from the foods you eat.[59] Keep that in mind when you are calculating how much water you have drank during the day when you are trying to make sure hydration needs are being met. There are also other fluids other than diuretics like soda, coffee, and alcohol that have water in them. Fruit juice is one, but as I previously mentioned I don't recommend drinking it since they're sugar havens. Milk is another fluid that has lots of water in it; approximately 87 percent of milk is water.[60]

Milk is a liquid that I don't tell people they can't have, but I do recommend you limit the amount of milk you drink. There is no added sugar in regular cow's milk, but there is some naturally occurring sugar (lactose) in milk.[61] You can rack up the calories by drinking milk pretty quick, especially if it's whole milk. Although, fat-free milk isn't as bad since it only contains 80 calories in a glass. The alcoholic drink Coffee Brandy with milk comes to mind. Coffee Brandy is a very popular drink in my home state of Maine. You'd be surprised how many calories you can suck down quickly drinking those bad boys. They add up fast and furiously.

I do want to point out the fact that milk is a decent source of protein. There are eight grams of high-quality protein in an eight-ounce glass, and plenty of calcium, which is why I say you don't need to avoid it altogether.[61] I do recommend you buy one percent rather than whole milk because whole milk has more fat in it. The one percent is lower in calories and, in my opinion, it doesn't taste much different than whole milk. Skim milk, on the other hand, tastes disgusting in my opinion, but if that's your choice of milk then go for it. I wouldn't drink much milk in a day, maybe a glass or just some with cereal in the morning is plenty. Want to know what, in my opinion, is better for you than cow's milk?

Almond milk (not the ones with added sugar like vanilla almond milk) is better for you than cow's milk, and it's lower in fat and calories. It doesn't have as much protein (one gram vs. eight grams in cow's milk), but it does have a good amount of other nutrients in it as well. Almond milk has about 45 percent of your daily value of calcium, as opposed to regular cow's milk at 30 percent. One thing that goes good with milk, or almond milk, are protein shakes.

Protein shakes are great if you are looking to build muscle or gain weight. I don't recommend you partake in protein shakes if you're looking to lose weight though. The kind of protein shakes I use and recommend are whey protein shakes. I buy the whey protein powder at Walmart, it's cheap, and it doesn't taste too bad if you mix it with just a little bit of milk. Whey protein is, in my opinion, the best quality protein shakes you can drink. However, don't take too much at one time. Your body can only process 30 grams of protein at a time in terms of muscle repair and building. Otherwise, anything more will likely be used as energy or stored as fat.[62]

Since protein shakes are a liquid protein, they digest much easier than if you eat something that's protein heavy, such as a steak. You can introduce 30 grams of protein into your bloodstream relatively quickly by drinking a protein shake. Eating the protein will cause a slower absorption, so if you were to eat more than 30 grams at a time it is likely most (if not all) of it is still usable for muscle repair and building, because of the slower digestion. If you are looking to gain weight or build muscle, you should try to consume about one gram of protein per pound of body weight a day.[63] If you do not seek to put on weight or build muscle, half the number of grams per pound of body weight will do.[3] Another kind of drink that I think is ok to drink is homemade fruit and or veggie smoothies.

I do not recommend drinking store bought smoothies as they contain extra, unneeded sugars or sweeteners, or they're made with fruit juice. Natural fruit smoothies you can make right at home are plenty sweet enough; there is no reason to add extra sugar or fruit juice to them. Fruit or veggie smoothies without any extra sugars or fruit juice are excellent for you. You can add protein to smoothies too by adding things like peanut butter, milk, or a scoop or two of protein powder. Homemade smoothies are excellent, tasty, and nutritious drinks that are awesome alternatives to drinking store bought smoothies loaded with extra sugar. Finally, if you follow all of these hydration rules that I've laid out for you, then it can have an enormous impact on your health and how you feel. The most important rule to remember in this chapter is, of course, rule number one; always stay hydrated.

Chapter Eight Summary:

- **Staying hydrated is so important for many reasons. Every chemical reaction in your body requires water to function properly. Your metabolism can't operate at peak efficiency if you're dehydrated and it can make you feel tired and sluggish.**

- **If you lose just one percent of your body's water, your mental performance and physical coordination begin to suffer. You start to feel thirsty if you have lost just two to three percent of your body's water.**

- **The human body is made up of anywhere from 60 to 75 percent water. Different factors affecting this number are age, gender, how much fat you carry around, or how lean you are.**

- **If you are properly hydrated and drinking the right fluids, you can feel better and more energetic, and your digestive system will thank you for it by functioning better than if you are dehydrated.**

- There are numerous benefits to water. If you drank just water for nine days straight, you could lose weight faster. Drinking just water for nine days is the equivalent of jogging over half a mile every day because of reduced calorie consumption from fluids.

- Staying hydrated can help you concentrate. The human brain is made up of 75 to 85 percent water.

- Water fills your belly, which can lead to appetite suppression, which subsequently can lead to weight loss.

- Water flushes out harmful toxins, which can help slow the aging process.

- Drinking plenty of water can lower the risk of many diseases ranging from hypertension (high blood pressure) to bladder conditions, and bowel cancer.

- Just five glasses of water a day can reduce the chance of a heart attack by up to 41 percent.

- Water helps to clear and moisten your skin, making your skin softer and cleaner.

- The standard eight, eight-ounce glasses of water a day should be ignored. No two bodies are identical in hydration needs.

- H_2O needs depends on three variables: weight, activity level, and climate. The more you weigh, the more active you are, the hotter or dryer the climate you live in, or a combination of any or all of these will mean an increase in your hydration needs.

- Take your weight and divide it in half and that is your base hydration needs in ounces. Example: if you are 200 pounds then you should drink a minimum of 100 ounces of water a day. The more active you are and the hotter or drier the climate you live in, the closer your hydration needs will go to one ounce of water per pound of body weight.

- A full cold glass of water first thing in the morning will give you a small, temporary metabolic boost and will help wake you up.

- The leaner you are, the more water you need to drink. Muscle contains more water than fat.

- The feeling of hunger isn't always directly caused by actual hunger. The same area of the brain that controls hunger controls thirst as well. Reach for some water first if there aren't obvious reasons why you feel hungry.

- In most cases, Gatorade is an unneeded sugary drink. Unless you are sweating profusely, you don't need a Gatorade. You can make an electrolyte drink like Gatorade without the added sugar right at home, don't waste your money and consume extra sugar with Gatorade.

- Soda is evil; tons of sugar (basically liquid sugar with some additives), caffeine, and it's a diuretic, meaning you pee out more than you would if you just drank plain water. Reduce or eliminate this horrible fluid.

- Soda calories or any liquid calories from anything but pure water can rack up quick. Be mindful of this when choosing your drinks.

- Even the old cliché of drinking ginger ale when you are sick is bad advice. Ginger ale has sugar in it just like any other soda. Even though ginger can soothe an upset stomach, you don't need to drink ginger ale to get ginger into your system.

- Diet soda is bad too. The sweetener aspartame and other junk they put in diet soda are horrible for you. If you are to drink soda, just plain old real sugar filled sodas are better for you. Best bet though is not to drink diet or regular soda, ever.

- A thing about coffee: it has health benefits in moderation. It's the creamer and sugar that's not good for you, not the coffee itself; as long as you don't drink too much of it. Black is the best way to drink coffee without adding extra calories and junk with sugar and creamer.

- Coffee does what people drink it for, it wakes you up, but it does more than just that. It gives your metabolism a temporary jolt, and can also give your memory a boost and give you better mental acuity.

- Too much coffee is bad because of excessive caffeine and its effects on sleep, and the fact that it's a diuretic.

- Limit alcohol consumption. Hangovers are caused by dehydration because alcohol is a diuretic.

- Alcohol in moderation does have some health benefits. Example: red wine is good for the heart, in moderation.

- The standard recommendation of no more than one glass for women and men over the age of 65 and two for men 65 and younger is a good rule of thumb. It certainly is ok to let loose now and then though.

- Limit or eliminate fruit juice altogether. Although fruit juice does have some nutritional value, unlike things like soda, it is also loaded with sugar without the fiber that comes with whole fruits.

- It is better to eat a whole fruit that has fiber in it that will slow the sugar absorption down than drinking fruit juice.

- Fruit juice contains more sugar and calories than whole fruit because, typically a glass of fruit contains the sugars from multiple pieces of fruit rather than just one whole piece of fruit.

- Sugar from fruit is naturally occurring; meaning it is not refined sugar like what you see in table sugar you put in coffee, cereal, etc. This means that even though yes, it is sugar, it is better for you. Remember to eat fruit which comes with fiber rather than drink your fruits though.

- If you are eating correctly, and especially if you load up on fruits and veggies, about 20 percent of your water needs are met through eating foods that contain water. Many fruits have a good amount of water in them.

- Limit the amount of milk you drink in a day. A glass a day or some with cereal in the morning is plenty. Calories from fluids like milk can add up rather quickly. This is why you should limit all types of fluid other than water.

- Milk is a good source of protein and things like calcium.

- Almond milk is better for you than regular cow's milk, in my opinion. Not as much protein (one gram as opposed to eight grams per an eight ounce glass), but a good source of other nutrients like calcium, which it contains more of than cow's milk.

- Protein shakes are great for building muscle or gaining weight, but I don't recommend them if you are trying to lose weight.

- Whey protein shakes are the best quality shakes.

- Don't consume too much protein in one sitting. Your body can't process more than 30 grams of protein at a time in terms of muscle repair and building. Excess protein is used as energy or stored as fat. Since protein shakes are a liquid form of protein, they digest quicker and easier than if you ate protein.

- If you're looking to gain weight or build muscle, you should try to be consuming about one gram of protein per pound of body weight, half that if you do not seek to gain weight or build muscle.

- Homemade fruit or vegetable smoothies are excellent alternatives to fruit juices as long as you do not add any unneeded sugars.

- Remember hydration rule number one: always stay hydrated.

Chapter Nine: *Implosion Leads to Belly Explosion*

Lesson 9: Putting too much pressure on yourself to be perfect all the time leads to certain failure.

What eventually happens to something you apply too much inward pressure to? It caves. If you squeeze a can hard enough it will cave inward. I believe humans operate in a similar manner. You can only apply so much pressure on yourself before you eventually implode. Striving for perfection is great. However, if you fail to be perfect you need to realize that you are only human, and it's impossible to be perfect all the time. You do not need to repeatedly put pressure on yourself to be spot on with your diet 100 percent of the time, or anything really. That's just not realistic. I am very guilty of making this blunder in the past, so I know that it's not good for your mental health to pressure yourself into being perfect 100 percent of the time. It will never happen, and when you do fail with that kind of pressure on yourself it can be devastating.

Everyone has their limits, whether we like to admit it or not. In the case of putting too much pressure on yourself while dieting, once you cave into the pressures of being spot on all the time, usually that will lead to binge eating.[64] You end up wanting to eat more of the unhealthy foods you're craving, and unless you have superhuman willpower and you can strong arm your way through the intense cravings for unhealthy foods, then you're going to give in eventually. Don't focus on being perfect 100 percent of the time.

You certainly don't want to stress yourself out if you fall short of perfection now and again. Stress can lead to weight gain.[65] Stress is not good for your health, both physically and mentally, and it can mess with your hormones.[65] You do not want your hormones out of whack, especially if you're trying to lose weight. The very thing you worry the most about can come true simply by putting too much stress on yourself. If you worry less, focus on doing the best you can, and jump back on the saddle if you fall off (but don't beat yourself up for it) then your goals are that much more within your grasp.

As long as you are great with your diet at least 80 percent of the time, then you're doing well enough that your diet should have a noticeable impact on your body and health. It's called the 80-20 rule.[3] A cheat meal here and there will not derail your success. In fact, thinking long-term, it can be beneficial to allow yourself to have a cheat meal now and again. Relieving pressure once in a while can help you to continually start over fresh with renewed strength towards your commitment to dieting the right way, which in turn can contribute to staving off binge eating. Binge eating is terrible for your diet, and it often leads to even more binge eating; this can have a domino effect. You want to avoid this at all costs. The 80-20 rule also applies to the connection of diet and exercise in how each one affects your looks.

All in all, constant perfection does not exist. As much as we may strive for that, and as close as we may come, we are imperfect beings and we live in an imperfect world; but there is hope. Eventually, over time, you can re-train your taste buds so that more healthy foods taste better and you don't crave something like sugar so badly. Your cravings for sugar can dissipate with a lot of time and patience. I know, I've been there; just give it time and effort.

Chapter Nine Summary:

- **All things that have too much inward pressure applied to them eventually cave. It's the same with us humans and our dieting.**

- **Putting too much pressure on yourself to be perfect all the time means there is a high chance of you eventually giving in and binge eating, which is one of the worst things you can do for your diet.**

- **Avoid stressing yourself out too much if you fall off the saddle. Stress is not good for your mental and physical health, and it can throw your hormones out of whack. None of which is conducive to reaching your goals, especially if that includes weight loss.**

- The 80-20 rule states that if you are good with your diet at least 80 percent of the time, then that is good enough for your diet to have a positive impact on your body and health.

- Allowing yourself a cheat meal now and again can relieve mental pressure from trying to be spot on with your diet all the time, which in turn can help stave off binge eating.

- Constant perfection does not exist, but it is possible to re-train your taste buds over time. This will cause more healthy foods to taste better, and your cravings for sugar to dissipate.

Chapter Ten: *Fad's Fade Away*

Lesson 10: If it's not a diet you can do for your entire life then it's a waste of time and energy.

The best results from dieting will always be achieved when you are doing things that will have long-term effects. Thinking short-term will only result in, you guessed it, short-term results. The advice I always give someone when they're planning on starting a new diet is this; stay away from fad diets. If the diet plan you are about to embark on isn't something that you can do for the rest of your life, then don't bother wasting your time doing it at all because there's a very high chance it will not give you long-term results. You need to always be thinking long-term. There are no shortcuts to success; lasting results take time, effort, and patience. Although, I will admit that the patience part has always been the most challenging aspect for me.

When someone starts a fad diet, what happens most often is that they may have some success with it, but once they start eating normally again it backfires. They may even lose some weight and feel good for a while, but it doesn't last and they may gain more weight in the end. Some fad diets are too strict, in my opinion. They leave you feeling tired and hungry. How good are your chances of success if you have to constantly battle those feelings? Also, fad diets usually ask you to cut out all kinds of food, sometimes unnecessarily.

I've known people who think that eating fruit when going on a low carb or no sugar diet is bad because of the sugar that is contained in fruits. That's completely false. Load up on fruits. Eat bowls full of fruit if you want to, just not the kind from a can which include all kinds of syrup that you do not need. Fruit is plenty sweet with a good amount of natural sugar, there is no need to add extra sugar with your fruit. You should also eat fruits because there's lots of water in fresh fruit, and it comes right along with fiber that will slow down the absorption of sugar into your blood stream. The fiber is what helps to prevent the sugar from digesting too quickly into the blood stream, which can cause a sugar spike.

Don't worry at all about how many carbs are in fruits or veggies because they contain complex carbs rather than the simple carbs that you get from junk food or refined and unnatural sugar. If you decide to do a low carb/high protein diet it doesn't mean you should cut out fruits and veggies, but simple carbs from junk food and limiting other carby foods. Simple carbs are quickly absorbed and can lead to sugar spikes and weight gain; complex carbs digest slowly, which helps to keep your blood sugar levels stable.[3] A blood sugar level that's stable is crucial for your weight.[3] I have personally seen people avoid fruit in favor of fatty meat because they think the sugar or carbs in fruit are going to slow down or halt their weight loss, or that they need to be consuming the protein instead. This is insanity, and completely the opposite of what you should be doing for the sake of your health. Yes, eat plenty of protein, but never think that eating some fruit is counterproductive to your weight loss journey, because that is so far from the truth.

With as carb conscious as the U.S. has become, it seems that some avoid carbs like it's the plague. I think this is why some fad diets have become so popular in recent years. I want to point out that it's not that you can't lose weight by going super skimpy on carbs, because you can; many people have. The science has been proven that yes, if you avoid carbs you can force your body to go into what's called ketosis.[66] In the interest of not getting too scientific, I'll break it down to the short version of what this means.

Ketosis means your body uses what's called ketones, and you are tricking your body into burning fat since there are little to no carbs being introduced into your body.[66] When your body doesn't have enough carbohydrates to turn into glucose for your cells to use as energy, it is forced to burn fat.[66] Although, too many ketones in your body can lead to what's called ketoacidosis. This is a very dangerous condition that results from ketones building up in your blood and becoming acidic. Ketoacidosis can ultimately lead to a coma or death.[3] As long as you don't go too far with ketosis, it's perfectly fine, but replacing fruits for more fatty meat for a lengthy amount of time is just simply not a healthier choice.

You see, many diet plans give you a short phase of going skimpy on the veggies and even skipping out on fruits to help go super low on carbs. This in the short-term is fine, but some take it way too extreme and think carbs will destroy their diet long after this initial phase. In the meanwhile, they're missing out on all kinds of vital nutrients and antioxidants found in fruits and veggies that aren't being eaten in place of meats; many times just any old fatty meat. Of course, not everyone goes crazy on fatty meat when their diet plan tells them to eat as much meat as they want while skipping on the fruits and going sparse on the veggies because of the carbs. This does happen quite often though, and I think it's a huge mistake and unnecessary.

A diet or weight loss plan should not just be about pure weight loss. Any weight loss program you choose to partake in should also coincide with what's best for your health. And any weight loss you seek can undoubtedly be attained by a diet that includes loading up on fruits and veggies with all their good carbs. I know this first hand. I have never cut out fruits or vegetables from my diet at any time, ever. And I have on several occasions been able to lose weight after coming back from a time when I have slipped and let myself go with a lack of exercise and poor diet. I've had to correct myself many times before for the sake of my health and waistline, but it never included cutting fruits and veggies. Still, I have always had success losing weight when I've made an honest attempt at it with a balanced and sensible diet and physical activity, without fail.

If you are considering a diet plan with the "all the meat you want to eat" mentality, let me ask you which is healthier, a barbecue or a salad? What about a barbecue vs. a fruit salad? What are the healthiest options? I think we all know the barbecue loses in both scenarios. A typical bbq is filled with all kinds of fatty meat and other fatty foods loaded with saturated fat and cholesterol. Burgers come to mind. Fruits and veggies, on the other hand, are filled with nutrients, antioxidants, and are low in calories. Now, I'm not saying don't eat meat. You can eat meat, just be sensible with your meat intake. There are better choices than just any old meat, and the "eat all you want" mentality of some diet plans. Opt for leaner meats like turkey, for example.

I don't advocate avoiding meat, but I'm not against vegetarianism either because you can obtain protein through other means than just meat. With all that being said, I won't argue the fact that yes, you can lose weight by cutting out carbs. However, you can also succeed in losing weight by eating healthy, low-calorie foods like fruits and veggies, other choices from the other food groups, and of course by physical activity. The dilemma is what's best for your overall health, rather than just what can cause the numbers on the scale to drop. You can lose weight by starving yourself as well, but we know without a doubt that's not the best and healthiest way to go about it. I feel the same about diet plans that encourage massive meat consumption in favor of light fruits and veggies. With some meats, preferably leaner meat choices, and some foods from all the major food groups across the board you can achieve a healthy mix of nutrients, and lose weight.

In the end, fad diets are just that, they are fads, and fads never last. Don't worry about being trendy when it comes to your diet, worry about doing things the right way. Wouldn't it be better for you to get results slowly, but results that stick around? Stay far, far away from diet plans or diet products that promise you a crazy amount of weight loss in a short period of time. These are hurting your chances of long-term success, and they are hurting your wallet. They are a waste of time and money. Seek out the better, slow path rather than a quick shortcut. You will see far better results in the end with long-term actions, and your health and body will thank you for it.

Chapter Ten Summary:

- **Long-term vs. short-term thinking and actions give you its equivalent in results.**

- Stay far away from fad diets. They are a waste of time and rarely will yield you long-term success.

- If a certain diet plan isn't something you can do for the rest of your life, or it's too strict, then there's no need to start it.

- There are no shortcuts to success; it takes time, effort, and patience.

- Some fad diets are too strict, leading you to short-term success followed by the regaining of weight loss, and sometimes additional weight gain.

- Some fad diets leave you feeling tired and hungry. Constantly battling those feelings makes it nearly impossible to succeed long-term.

- If eating a low carb, high protein diet, don't forsake fruit because of the sugar in it. Sugar from fruit is natural and you consume it with fiber, which slows down sugar absorption, helping to prevent sugar spikes.

- Complex carbs from fruits and veggies can be consumed in abundance. A low carb diet should not restrict fruits and vegetables, but simple carbs from junk food and other non-fruits and veggies products.

- Simple carbs lead to sugar spikes and possible weight gain. Complex carbs absorb slowly and help keep blood sugar levels stable.

- Eat plenty of protein, but also fruits and veggies. Do not choose fatty meat over fruit just because there's sugar in fruit. This is entirely the wrong line of thinking for your health and weight.

- You do not need to avoid carbs like the plague. Eating too few carbs can lead to ketosis, which does cause your body to burn fat, but too many ketones in your body can become acidic and lead to ketoacidosis; which can lead to a coma or even death.

- Avoiding fruits or going very light on veggies in favor of just any old fatty meat, and as much meat as you want as some diets encourage, is not, in my opinion, the healthiest path to weight loss.

- Some diet plans give you a phase of little to no carbs, including carbs from fruits or veggies. These are typically short-term, which is fine, but some take it way too extreme and avoid carbs long after the initial phase, the thought being that carbs will destroy their diet.

- Extreme low carb dieting usually means missing out on healthy nutrient and antioxidant-dense fruits and veggies in favor of meats, often fatty meats.

- A diet or weight loss plan should not just purely be about losing weight, but it should also coincide with what is best for your health during the weight loss process.

- Any weight loss you seek can without a doubt be obtained while still loading up on fruits and vegetables.

- If you are considering an "all the meat you want to eat" mentality of a diet plan, then first think of a barbecue vs. salad, or fruit salad. Barbecue loses in both scenarios. Bbq's are typically filled with fatty meats and other fatty foods. Fruits and vegetables are loaded with nutrients, antioxidants, and are low in calories.

- I'm not against eating meat, but be sensible with meat intake; opt for leaner meats, such as turkey, for example. I'm not against vegetarianism either; protein can be obtained through other means rather than just meat.

- It is a fact that you can lose weight by cutting carbs way down, but you can also accomplish weight loss by still eating nutritious fruits and vegetables. The dilemma is what is best for your health, not just any old plan that will drop the number on the scale. You can lose weight by starving yourself too, but we know that's not the best path. The same can be argued against any heavy meat eating plans vs. balanced diets that include fruits and vegetables.

- A healthy mix of nutrients from all food groups is the best course of action for diet, including weight loss.

- Fad diets fade away. It's better to achieve results slowly, but results that will stick around, rather than to look for shortcuts that fade away just like the fad diet.

- Avoid products or diet plans that promise an insane amount of weight loss can be accomplished in a short period of time. Seek out the better, slow path and you will see better results in the end. Your health and body will thank you for it as well.

Chapter Eleven: *Track It or Lose It*

Lesson 11: Write all your diet progress and actions down.

A common kitchen blunder I see people make is not tracking the things they need to pay attention to in order to see where they are headed. If you want diet success, plus the success of whatever goals you have along with that, you should be tracking all relevant factors. Unless you have superior memory skills you should be writing down everything from your body weight, body fat, and body measurements. I also highly recommend keeping a food journal, particularly in the beginning of a new diet. Over time you can train your brain to remember everything you eat in a day because it will become habitual. Until it becomes routine and you can track it in your mind you should be writing down in a journal every little piece of food that goes into your mouth. You truly won't know how much you're eating unless you track it.

We've already talked about weighing yourself and taking body fat and body measurements once a week, but remember to write it all down too. Tracking your food intake by writing it all down will help you tremendously with your diet. Besides, how do you know where you are going if you're not tracking where you've been? I'm a bit of a perfectionist, so I advocate doing things as perfectly as possible. Obsessing over the right things is not a bad thing.

The most successful people on the planet are obsessive. They just obsess over the things that drive them towards success. Think of someone like Steve Jobs. He was obsessed with his company and what needed to be done to win. Think of Arnold Schwarzenegger. That man was obsessed about bodybuilding; I mean really obsessed. I don't say that in a bad way at all. It truly takes that kind of commitment to have enormous success if you want to be the best. Arnold wouldn't have had the success that he did if he had haphazardly tried to be a champion bodybuilder. No way, never would have happened. Steve Jobs would not have created one of the greatest companies on the planet, Apple, if he had not been obsessed with winning and being the best. I'm not saying that you have to become so obsessive with your diet everything else in your life becomes secondary, but if you want to have extreme results sometimes it takes extreme measures. Now, a food journal is a great tool you can use to track what you're consuming if you want some serious success.

A food journal will often surprise people. Generally, people tend to underestimate how much food or how many calories they are eating in the course of a day; sometimes grossly so. When first starting a diet or trying to lose weight, write down every little thing you eat. When you first start a new diet that is when a food journal is the most important. A food journal helps you spot trends or places you need to adjust to make your diet effective. It also helps to hold yourself accountable. Accountability is imperative. Unless you were to have someone with you all day to slap your hand every time you reached for some crummy food you need something to help keep yourself honest, such as a food journal.

Food journal aside, at the very least you should stop and think before anything touches your mouth. Ask yourself this: is what I'm about to eat going to put me closer to my goals and the body of my dreams, or pull me further away? Should you enjoy that piece of cheesecake that will give you pleasure for five minutes, or work to achieve the body of your dreams? Everything that you eat you ultimately choose to put it into your body. Make the right choices and I guarantee you'll stand a far better chance of reaping the benefits of good health and a great body. Stopping to think before you eat can develop into an excellent habit over time. You see, we humans are naturally habitual creatures. If you can develop good habits and eliminate bad ones, how on earth are you ever going to fail?

The most successful people in the world, no matter what area of life it is in (business, relationships, fitness, or whatever) are not only obsessive, but they also have "successful" habits.

They develop and maintain these success habits. These are simply things they do on a daily basis that moves them towards a meaningful goal. Some examples of habits you can develop that will make it highly likely that your diet is going to be hugely successful are things we have already discussed; always eat breakfast, always eat a protein with every meal, keep portions a reasonable size, maintain a food journal, etc. Some bad habits that we have also discussed are things like eating too late at night, or too close to bed, not consuming enough vegetables, grabbing a sugar filled coffee on the way to work, etc. Remember to develop the right habits, and one of them should be to track everything. It's fun when you start to see progress, and you've got written proof of it.

Chapter Eleven Summary:

- **Unless you have superior memory skills, track everything including your body weight, body fat, body measurements, and food consumption by writing it down. A** food journal is a handy device for tracking your food intake.

- Until it becomes habitual in your mind, write every little thing you eat down. You truly won't know how much you're eating unless you track it.

- Being obsessive about the right things, like tracking your food intake, is not a bad thing. The most successful people on the planet are obsessive about doing what it takes to be the best.

- A food journal often surprises people when they can see how much they are truly eating in a day. People tend to underestimate how much they eat.

- A food journal helps to keep yourself honest and accountable.

- Stop to think before eating: is this food going to put me closer to my goals, or further away. Thinking like this can develop into an excellent habit. Developing good habits and eliminating bad ones will put you within the realm of success.

- The most successful people on the planet are not only obsessive, but they develop and maintain excellent success habits that drive them towards a meaningful goal.

- Develop healthy diet habits, like never skipping breakfast, eating a protein with every meal, keeping portions reasonable, maintaining a food journal, etc.

- Eliminate bad habits, such as eating too late at night or too close to bedtime, not eating enough vegetables, grabbing a sugar filled coffee on the way to work, etc.

- Tracking everything is a success habit, and it's fun when you start seeing results, and you have written proof of it.

Chapter Twelve: *The Grocery List*

Lesson 12: A collection of helpful tips and useful knowledge.

The lessons in this book have predominantly been about diet mistakes you need to avoid if you want to achieve optimal results for your health and your physique. This section of the book goes further by focusing on tidbits of useful information that you will find very helpful when working towards your diet goals. This collection of useful knowledge will round out this guide, so that you have all the necessary information that you need to achieve the absolute best diet results possible. Here is the "Grocery List" of tips and useful knowledge.

The Food Groups:

Here is a list of all the different kinds of the main food groups (meats, vegetables, fruits, grains, dairy, and healthy fats) and some tips and advice regarding each one. This list also includes information on typical serving sizes for each food group. The amount of servings you need per group is based on your specific calorie needs as it pertains to your goals. The best way to figure out how many servings per food group you need is to know what percentage of calories you need from each group, and how many calories are in all the different foods you eat within each food group. I've laid all this out for you in this section as well to assist you in your meal planning.

All in all, it's better to worry about portion control and how many calories you're eating from each food group than to count servings, but servings are an important way to measure and track how many calories you are consuming from all the different foods you're eating. Finally, remember this rule; balance is key. Balance is what you should always be seeking. A well-balanced diet will always be what is best for your health, and it's good for the waistline.

Percentages of Food Groups: The biggest portion of a well-balanced diet should consist of mostly fruits, vegetables, and some whole grains. Roughly 45 to 60 percent of the calories you consume in your diet should comprise of these major food groups, with vegetables being the most consumed, fruits second most, and then some grains.[67] Calories from proteins should equal roughly 10 to 35 percent of your diet.[67] Remember that protein can come from other sources other than meat, such as beans and nuts. Finally, calories from healthy fats should comprise of anywhere from about 25 to 35 percent of your daily caloric intake.[67] You should also include one or two servings of dairy a day.[3]

Meats: A good rule of thumb when it comes to what is considered a serving size of meat is that one serving (three ounces cooked) is approximately the size of a deck of cards. This is a rough guess that's usually pretty close to what a serving size should be. If you want to get technical, you could always get a scale that measures food weight, but if you don't already have one it's not crucial that you be that tedious with measuring your food. But, if you want to do that it certainly won't hurt, it would only help you. There's not much that I suggest you shouldn't eat, but of course, eat in moderation. Certainly go light with meats that are high in saturated fat, such as beef.

When shopping, I recommend you buy the leanest meats you can find. If you're buying beef, buy the leanest cut you can find. Turkey is my number one pick for meat. It is one of the leanest meats you can eat. Also, keep in mind that white meat generally contains fewer calories and fat than dark meat.[68] I recommend eating skinless chicken. Eggs are the best source of protein you can eat because they contain plenty of amino acids right along with the protein, which is needed for your body to utilize the protein.[69] Eat plenty of fish, such as salmon, tilapia, and tuna. These are excellent choices in fish. And remember that many fish are usually a good source of omega-3 fatty acids, which is essential for brain health.[70]

Here is a list of meats that I recommend in order from best to worst:

1. Turkey
2. Chicken (skinless)
3. Eggs (best source of meat protein)
4. Salmon
5. Tilapia
6. Tuna
7. Lamb
8. Pork
9. Beef

Veggies: It's typically better to steam most vegetables than to boil them. Boiling them will cause nutrient leaching.[71] I will touch on this later in the cooking methods section of this chapter. I buy veggie steamers at Walmart; they're good and super simple to cook. You can also opt to eat your vegetables raw and save time and energy on cooking them, and it's a healthy option. Not to beat a dead horse, but eat as many veggies as you please; it's tough to eat too much of these. A serving of vegetables is one cup of raw, leafy vegetables or ½ cup of other kinds of veggies. A serving size is normally about the size of a small fist.

Here's a list of some great veggies that I recommend you mix into your diet (alphabetized list):

1. Artichoke
2. Arugula
3. Asparagus
4. Aubergine (eggplant)
5. Legumes (pretty much any kind of bean, which are also a good source of protein)
6. Beet greens
7. Broccoli
8. Brussels sprouts
9. Cabbage
10. Carrots
11. Cauliflower
12. Celery
13. Chard
14. Collard greens
15. Fiddleheads (these are delicious, in my opinion)
16. Herbs and spices (feel free to load up on any of these, and they're great for adding taste.)
17. Kale

18. Lettuce
19. Mushrooms
20. Mustard greens
21. Onions (any kind)
22. Parsley
23. Peppers (any kind, green, red, etc.)
24. Radish (any kind)
25. Root vegetables (any kind, ginger is an excellent choice)
26. Spinach (Good source of protein too)
27. Squash (Any kind)
28. Tomato
29. Tubers (the thick part of a stem plant that have buds from which new plants can grow. Potatoes are tubers. I recommend eating any kind. Sweet potatoes fall into this category as well as white potatoes. Yam is a tuber too)[72]
30. Turnip greens
31. Water chestnut
32. Watercress
33. Zucchini.

Fruits: Eat less fruit than veggies, but you can eat these generously. Even if you only eat fruits for a snack, and maybe sometimes with a meal, that's plenty of fruit servings in a day. One medium sized fruit, or a ½ cup of chopped or canned fruit, is considered one serving. One medium sized fruit is about the size of a baseball.

Here is a list of some great fruits I recommend you mix into your diet (alphabetized list):

1. Apple
2. Apricot
3. Avocado (good source of healthy fat too)[73]
4. Banana
5. Blackberry
6. Blueberry (considered a super fruit and might be the healthiest fruit you can eat.)[74]
7. Cherry
8. Coconut
9. Cranberry
10. Cucumber
11. Date
12. Dragon fruit
13. Fig
14. Goji berry
15. Grapes (raisins too, which is a dried grape.)
16. Guava
17. Honeyberry
18. Huckleberry

19. Kiwi
20. Kumquat
21. Lemon
22. Lime
23. Mango
24. Melon (all kinds, watermelon, cantaloupe, etc.)
25. Orange
26. Papaya
27. Peach
28. Pear
29. Plum
30. Pineapple
31. Pomegranate (considered a super fruit like blueberries)[75]
32. Raspberry
33. Star fruit (carambola)
34. Strawberry
35. Pumpkin

Grains: Whole grains are the best kind of grains, and most grains do have a whole grain option, like bread for example. Limit sugary and refined grains. I absolutely would not eat white bread; it's unhealthy in my opinion. In the interest of not eating too many carbs, I would not go heavy on grains like you can with fruits and veggies, but you can eat some in moderation. Whole grains are the best option because they digest slower than refined grains, which help to keep blood sugar levels in check.[76] Because of this, eating whole grains in place of refined options may help to prevent type II diabetes, heart disease, stroke, and they may even help lower blood pressure.[77] Typically, whole grains also contain more nutrients than refined options.[76] One serving of grains is one slice of bread, an ounce of ready-to-eat cereal, or ½ cup of rice or pasta. A typical serving is about ½ the size of a baseball.

Here is a list of grains I recommend you can eat (alphabetized list):

1. Amaranth
2. Barley
3. Brown Rice
4. Buckwheat
5. Bulgar (cracked wheat)
6. Farro/Emmer
7. Flaxseed
8. Grano
9. Millet
10. Oats (oat bread, oat Cereal, oatmeal)
11. Popcorn (go light with the salt and butter)

12. Whole wheat cereal flakes
13. Muesli
14. Rolled oats
15. Quinoa
16. Rye
17. Sorghum
18. Spelt
19. Teff
20. Triticale
21. Whole grain barley
22. Wheat berries
23. Whole rye
24. Whole wheat bread
25. Whole wheat couscous
26. Whole wheat crackers
27. Whole wheat pasta
28. Whole wheat pita bread
29. Whole wheat sandwich buns and rolls
30. Whole wheat tortillas
31. Wild rice

Refined Grains: Go light on these.

1. Crackers
2. Flour tortillas
3. Grits
4. Noodles
5. Spaghetti
6. Macaroni

7. Pasta (limit these as they are carb heavy. It's not that carbs are evil, but too much of anything is bad)
8. Pitas
9. Pretzels
10. Ready to eat breakfast cereals

Healthy Fats Including Dairy: You don't have to cut out dairy as some would suggest, but do go light on it. I wouldn't drink more than a cup of milk a day (one serving), and eat cheese in moderation (1-1/2 ounces of cheese is one serving.) These are good sources of protein and do have nutritional benefits, but generally they are high in fat and can slow up digestion.[78] Also, approximately one teaspoon is considered a serving of fats and oils, which is about the equivalent of the tip of your thumb.

Dairy:

1. Milk (I recommend choosing a low-fat jug rather than whole milk. You don't need to choose skim milk; I personally find that disgusting. I buy the one percent, but skim is fine if that's your preference. However, I barely notice

any difference between one percent and whole milk, but that's just what my taste buds have to say.)

2.   Cheese (cottage cheese is really good for you and an excellent source of protein.)[79] Avoid or limit processed cheese. However, swiss, parmesan, string cheese, full-fat cheese, and feta are the healthiest choices along with cottage cheese.[80,81]

3.   Yogurt (I recommend Greek yogurt. These are good sources of protein. I find Greek yogurt that has some fat in it to be pretty tasty. The zero fat ones are disgusting, according to my taste buds. Yogurts that haven't had any fat removed from them are perfectly healthy for you. That and yogurts are good for your digestive system.)[82]

Healthy Fats Other Than Dairy: Some of these are listed and discussed elsewhere too, but for simplicity's sake here are my recommendations for healthy fats:

1.   Avocados

2. Dark chocolate
3. Whole Eggs (I never recommend just egg whites like a lot of health "gurus" do. The yolk is good for you and a healthy fat.)[83]
4. Fatty fish (fish like salmon, trout, mackerel, sardines, and herring. As I previously mentioned, these are loaded with heart and brain healthy omega-3 fatty acids, and they're a good source of protein.)
5. Nuts (these are very healthy; they are high in healthy fats, fiber, and protein.)[87]
6. Chia seeds
7. Extra virgin olive oil
8. Coconuts and coconut oil
9. Full fat yogurt

Cooking Methods:

There are plenty of healthy ways to cook food without the need to add unnecessary extras. However, I do not recommend frying food, or at least do it sparingly. The frying process adds boatloads of calories and fat to food because of the need to use oil or fat to fry it up.[85] You can limit the amount of fat or oil added to the food to a degree, but regardless, frying simply isn't the healthiest cooking method. Baking is a better option than frying because you don't need to add fats and oils to cook the food.[86] The frying process can also rob foods of some of their nutritional value.[87] Also, keep in mind when eating out that many restaurants prepare foods with unhealthy hydrogenated oils that have unhealthy trans fats in them.[85]

Trans fats are the worst kinds of fats and are linked to clogged arteries and heart disease.[88] I strongly recommend you severely limit trans fats from your diet. Healthy fats like olive oil have just the opposite effect that trans fats have on the body. They can help lower your risk of heart disease and even remove cholesterol from your blood stream.[89] However, you should still eat these healthy fats in moderation, as they are high in calories. Also, I want to point out that the three primary macronutrients (fats, carbs, and protein) are measured in calories per gram. A fat gram is worth nine calories, carbs and protein are worth four calories per gram. This is important to know when tracking calorie intake.

It's important to know when choosing which cooking method to use that heat can break down and destroy up to 15 to 20 percent of vitamins in vegetables.[90] Destruction of vitamins from heat is particularly the case when it comes to vitamin C, folate, and potassium.[90] Some say that for this reason, it's best to eat foods raw when possible to retain all of the food's nutritional value.[90] However, some studies have shown that cooking can be beneficial for some foods. For example, carrots, spinach, and tomatoes release antioxidants when heated, causing a breakdown of the food's cell walls, which makes it easier for the human body to absorb them.[90] Antioxidants (mostly found in plant-based foods or drinks) are elements you undeniably want to include in your diet.

Antioxidants are substances that prevent or completely stop cells from being damaged by oxidants.[91] Oxidants are also known as free radicals that are found in the environment or produced naturally by our bodies.[92] Free radicals are created by normal cellular functions, but too many of them can cause serious damage and lead to things such as certain cancers and heart disease.[93] Oxidants also come from environmental substances such as air pollution, cigarette smoke, and medication.[93] With this being said though, don't overdo it on antioxidants, too many can suppress your body's ability to turn on its own antioxidant defense system.[94] This is another example of too much of a good thing turning into something not so good. So, knowing all this, what are the healthiest cooking methods? The healthiest options I recommend for cooking can range from steaming, boiling, microwaving, poaching, broiling, grilling, baking, or stir frying.[90] Other than baking, which I've already mentioned, the following ones that I've listed below are the methods I consider to be the healthiest options for cooking.

Steaming: This method of cooking allows foods like veggies to stew in their own juices, which in turn helps to retain a lot of their nutritional value.[90]

Boiling: This may be a better option over steaming with certain foods such as carrots, zucchini, and broccoli. Research has shown that boiling helps these foods retain their nutrients the most.[90] However, the high temps of boiling and the large amount of boiling water can dissolve and wash away water-soluble vitamins and up to 70 percent of minerals in some foods, especially certain vegetables.[90]

Microwaving: Surprisingly, this cooking method may be the healthiest way to cook because of the short cooking times. The shorter the cooking time, the fewer nutrients are destroyed by heat.[90] You can microwave almost anything and without the need to add extra calorie-dense oils.

Poaching: This method is similar to boiling but requires less water, and it takes longer to cook food this way. The longer cooking times with poaching may result in more nutrient destruction, but it's a great way to gently cook delicate foods like fish, or eggs.[90]

Broiling: This cooking method is a great way to cook tender cuts of meat, but not so much for cooking veggies. Broiling cooks food in high, direct heat very quickly.[90]

Grilling: This is a great option in that it doesn't require you to add all kinds of fats. However, eating charred, well-done meat on a regular basis can increase the risk of pancreatic and breast cancer, so don't do this regularly.[90]

Stir Frying: This method does require some cooking oil, but only a moderate amount.[90] This method is ideal for food like bite sized meats, grains such as rice and quinoa, and veggies that are thin-cut. Some examples of vegetables that would normally be thin cut are bell peppers, julienne carrots, and snow peas.[90]

Ingredient Lists:

Food manufacturers are required by law to give you nutritional information on their food labels.[95] When looking at labels, know that the ingredients are listed from most to least by weight.[96] For example, if the first ingredient on the package says sugar then that means that particular food contains more sugar than anything else. If the last ingredient is wheat then that means the food product has less wheat in it than anything else. Also, when reading ingredient lists, it's a good rule of thumb that if you don't know what an ingredient is or you can't pronounce it, then you probably shouldn't be eating it.

Food additives have all kind of impossible to pronounce names. Avoiding strange ingredients is extremely difficult given the fact that most American food is processed garbage, but do the best you can to find the most organic wholesome foods in the market. These are always pricier, but budget them into your diet the best you can. Often, if people cut out most or all of the junk in their diet it frees up enough of their budget that at least some organic foods can be bought. If you want to go a step further, invest in starting a garden, if you don't already have one. It's work, and it can save you money and reap you quality food in the process.

Carb Heaven:

Carb heaven is a term I like to use to categorize all the tasty but less than ideal foods that contain lots of simple carbs. These are the opposite of the kinds of foods that contain the good, complex carbs you get from foods like fruits and veggies. Foods of this nature should be the lowest priority in your diet. As I've said before, cheat meals here and there are ok, but stay light on carb heaven foods. These are what I feel are yummy foods like sweets or junk food. Things like pizza, baked goods, etc. also fall into this category. Carb Heaven is your health's road to hell, stay off Carb Heaven Highway.

Supplements:

If you are eating properly and plentifully there really shouldn't be any need for supplements. In my opinion, most supplements are not harmful, but they're a waste of money. Unless keeping a tight budget is not a necessity for you, there's really no reason to spend all kinds of money on supplements. The only times I recommend using some supplements is when you are going a bit extreme with your diet, or when you are trying to build a significant amount of muscle with your workouts.

If you are eating very lightly because of a diet you are on, it is likely you are going to end up a bit short in the vitamins and minerals category, so supplementing for those is not a bad idea. If you're pumping iron in the gym and want to pack on some muscle, you need to ingest lots of protein, so I recommend taking protein supplements such as protein shakes. Then again, this is only really necessary if you aren't consuming at least the recommended one gram of protein per pound of body weight.

If you are eating enough protein, then there's no need to buy extra protein supplements. However, in some rare cases you might need tons of protein, such as if you're a professional bodybuilder. Supplementing your protein in cases like these can save you money because if you supplement your protein, you don't need to eat as much food. When I'm doing a bodybuilding routine in the gym, I only buy protein powder to supplement my protein. That's it. I don't spend any money on anything else. I don't think it's necessary for the average person to spend extra money on all kinds of supplements. It may be a different story with someone like a professional bodybuilder who may need to go further with supplementation, but have you seen how much muscle those guys pack on? Also, think of prison inmates. A lot of those guys get huge while in prison, but I seriously doubt they have access to, or are smuggling in all kinds of supplements. They rely on strictly food and weights, and many of them build an enormous amount of muscle. Finally, it's not that supplements don't have their benefits, but unless your career is professional bodybuilding, I don't see a need for a cabinet full of supplements.

Salt and Pepper:

Salt, in the proper quantities, is necessary for your diet. Salt is needed for maintaining healthy functioning of your body's cells, nerve conduction, digestion, to help absorb nutrients, and to eliminate waste.[97] However, because too much sodium (the main ingredient of regular salt) is bad for blood pressure and water retention, I recommend going easy on table salt. The absolute maximum amount of sodium you can safely eat in a day is 2,300 milligrams.[98] If you do have table salt, make sure you use salt that has iodine in it, which is good for your thyroid.[98] The thyroid has direct control on your metabolism.[99] You want your thyroid to be able to operate at its most optimal levels.

Pepper, and other natural spices and herbs, can be used generously. In fact, pepper is good for your heart, so pour it right on if you so desire.[101] I love pepper; I pour that on and drive it right home. There is an ongoing debate about sea salt vs. regular table salt. Despite the fact that sea salt is commonly promoted as being healthier than table salt, they both have the same basic nutritional value, and both contain comparable amounts of sodium. The differences lie in their taste, texture, and processing.[98]

Sea salt, if the name doesn't give it away, comes from the sea. Table salt is usually mined from underground salt deposits.[98] Sea salt is not as heavily processed as table salt, which does leave trace amounts of minerals.[98] The minerals add flavor and color.[98] Table salt, on the other hand, is heavily processed, which eliminates minerals.[98] It also has an additive that helps to prevent clumping.[98] Regular salt also contains other unhealthy additives.[97] Most table salt does have iodine added to it though. A different kind of salt, which I consider to be a good replacement for regular salt, is Pink Himalayan salt.

Pink Himalayan salt is considered the cleanest and most beneficial salt on the planet today, and with good reason.[97] It is said to be over 99 percent pure.[97] This kind of salt contains a whopping amount of minerals and trace elements, 84 to be more precise.[97] It includes things like calcium, magnesium, potassium, copper, and iron.[97] These are all essential nutrients you need in your daily diet. Pink Himalayan salt also contains less sodium than regular salt.[97] Because regular salt is heavily processed, which eliminates minerals, it is made up of anywhere from 97.5 percent to 99 percent sodium chloride.[97] As I mentioned before, Himalayan salt is unrefined, and it only contains about 87 percent sodium chloride.[97] Pink Himalayan salt isn't just known for its nutritional benefits, but it is also known to have other health benefits as well.

Pink Himalayan salt is believed to have the ability to improve respiratory problems, balance your body's pH (good for digestion and immunity), it can help you sleep better, and has many other benefits as well.[97] Regardless of all these benefits, you still need to go light on any kind of salt because too much sodium causes problems. As I previously mentioned, the recommended amount of sodium in a day is less than 2,300 milligrams no matter which salt you choose to eat, but I think the Pink Himalayan salt is the superior choice.

Six Pack Abs:

The kitchen is your lab for making a set of six pack abs; the gym is the hammer and chisel where you make it a true work of body sculpting art. Diet plays the biggest part in achieving a set of six pack abs, which so many of us desire. To reveal a six pack, you just need to keep dieting and exercising until enough fat comes off that you can finally see your abs. For men, you need to bring your body fat percentage down below 10 percent before you start seeing your abs.[112] For women, you need to get your body fat percentage down below 13 percent.[112] These are general figures, as not everyone has the same genetic makeup and fat distribution.[112]

In general, most fat is stored in the gut area, especially for us dudes.[100] However, you cannot do what's called "spot reduction." You can't just pick where you want your body to burn fat.[102] Doing a bunch of sit-ups isn't going to target fat in your belly to be burned. Fat is lost according to your genetic makeup.[112] Generally, body fat is pulled from all over your body when you burn fat, and the gut is the last place to lose because of the fact that most fat is usually stored there.[112] If you are eating a well-balanced diet and you exercise regularly, a nice set of six pack abs is absolutely in the realm of possibility.

Variety Is the Spice of Life, and Your Diet:

An important tip to remember for the sake of your health is that you need to have not only a balanced diet, but a varied one too. Eating a variety of foods will ensure that you're getting the different kinds of vitamins and minerals your body needs. Our bodies are not designed to eat the same exact foods every day. Besides, that would get boring eating the same foods day in and day out.

"Eat the Rainbow":

This catchphrase simply means, eat a variety of fresh produce of different colors. The reason why you want to vary what color produce you eat is because the color indicates an abundance of a certain nutrient.[103] So, if you eat a variety of colors you are certain to get plenty of different nutrients your body needs. It's also important to "eat the rainbow" because not only can eating unhealthy foods lead to disease, but so can the absence of healthy foods from your diet. This is part of the reason for the enormous importance of fruits and veggies. They are not just good for the waistline, but as a bonus, they are health boosters too.

Dressings:

Overloading your food with dressing is relatively easy to do. I know, I've done it on many occasions. Lettuce definitely does taste a whole lot better when you drench it in ranch dressing, but I caution you to use dressings sparingly. You would be surprised to see how many extra calories you can add by using dressings on food that is low in calories; lowering the benefit of eating a low-calorie food, such as lettuce. There is an exception though; mustard has, quite literally, zero calories. So, drench away with the yellow, yummy goodness.

Vegetarianism:

I've never personally followed a vegetarian diet, but I do consider it a good choice for those who wish to follow a healthy lifestyle. The only thing I recommend if you want to try a vegetarian diet is to make sure you are still getting plenty of protein through other plant-based foods, since you won't be eating meat. Things like beans, nuts, and spinach are excellent sources of protein for a vegetarian diet.

Option A, B, Or:

Some foods have multiple versions of the same food. Here are a few examples of common foods and which versions I think are the best.

Potatoes: Both regular and sweet potatoes are good carbs, and contain nutritional value. Many believe sweet potatoes are better for you than regular potatoes. The fact is that they are similar in nutritional value, except sweet potatoes do have more sugar and a whole lot more vitamin A. Sweet potatoes also have slightly higher levels of certain other vitamins. I recommend eating both, but sweet potatoes for the narrow win. Also, you get more nutrients if you eat the skins of potatoes. However, if you peel them, make sure you peel thinly because most of the nutrients are close to the skin.

Rice: Brown rice or white rice? Brown rice is the obvious choice. Brown rice is a whole grain that contains what is called the bran and germ. Because of this, they provide fiber and many vitamins and minerals.[104] White rice is a refined grain that has had the nutritious parts removed. White rice is essentially "empty calories" and carbs with very little nutritional content.[104]

Cooking Spray: I highly recommend Smart Balance cooking spray over regular cooking spray like PAM, or even oil, which is pretty much pure fat. Smart Balance has much more nutritional value than other sprays and is generally lower in calories.

Butter: Smart Balance wins again. I recommend Smart Balance over regular butter or margarine. It's lower in calories and contains fewer bad fats. From what I've noticed, Smart Balance butter adds superior healthy fats such as omega-3 fatty acids, which helps boost the brain.

Cheese please: Some cheese is known to be high in fat and calories, so I don't recommend eating pounds of it, but it is a good source of protein and has other health benefits. So don't fret, I won't tell you that you can't enjoy this wonderful thing in life called cheese. Cheese is such a popular food that it would be difficult to write a nutritional book and not include a segment on cheese. Just like bacon, eat bacon if you so choose, just don't overdo it. Balance is a good general rule of thumb on virtually any food. Also, it's important to point out that the FDA has some strict regulations on what is considered cheese and what is not.

Anything that is processed cannot be sold as cheese, but has to be labeled a cheese product. This means it contains less than 51 percent cheese.[105] You want to stay away from processed cheese just as you do with any other kind of processed foods. To recap, the types of cheese I do recommend from the food groups section of this chapter are the following: cottage cheese (an excellent source of protein), swiss, parmesan, string cheese (yes string cheese), full-fat cheese, and feta.

There are several kinds of cheese I recommend you stay away from, some of them being low-fat cheese, and of course "cheese products." Also, anything that is labeled low sugar, or reduced fat, sugar, etc., you should steer clear from. The reason for this is because anytime naturally occurring ingredients are removed they are frequently replaced with harmful ingredients to make up for the lost flavor.[106] Reduced sodium cheddar is another cheese you should stay away from. When food is stripped of its natural ingredients, you need to ask yourself, what are substituting the ingredients that have been removed? Food manufacturers don't just remove stuff from food and leave it as is; it would leave the food inedible. Also, cheese that has added ingredients, like sweetened cream cheese, you should stay away from too. These usually have added harmful products that I have talked about previously, such as aspartame, which is known to cause gastrointestinal problems.[107]

Frozen Yogurt, or Ice Cream, or Maybe Pudding?:
Both frozen yogurt and ice cream are loaded with
sugar. However, if you are going to cheat then do it
wisely. Frozen yogurt is a better cheat option than
straight up ice cream. As much as I love ice cream,
typically, frozen yogurt does have less sugar, and
yogurt also has live and active cultures that you
won't find in plain old ice cream. So, when deciding
on the best cheating course of action, opt for frozen
yogurt. If you do opt for the more evil of the two
choices though, grab some slow churned ice cream.
Those versions have less fat in them, but taste just
as good as regular ice cream. My other favorite
cheat: pudding. This food also falls into what I like
to call, the class of cheaters. Believe it or not, you
can enjoy the foods you love now and again and still
meet your health and fitness goals. How exciting
could life be without the occasional cheat? However,
remember to indulge sparingly.

Emotional Eating:

One of the worst times to eat is when you are feeling emotional. I know for some, myself included, emotional eating can prove to be incredibly difficult to overcome. Food is comforting for many people, which is why you hear people sometimes refer to food as "comfort food." To curb this, you have no choice but to use your willpower to stop and think about what you are about to eat before indulging. Eat with your head, not your emotions. I believe that emotional eating is a huge link to obesity and other health problems associated with improper food intake. I am so very upsettingly guilty of emotional eating. I've blundered countless times eating emotionally rather than eating only to give my body the energy and proper nutrients it needs, but I have been able to overcome it as well.

What I suggest doing to prevent emotional eating is to find some way to distract your mind. The best way to do that, in my opinion, is to do something physical or do a workout, especially a cardio workout. Cardio is known to curb appetite, while lifting weights may stimulate hunger.[112] When you force your mind to focus on something else other than food to comfort the way you feel, you will have a much better chance of avoiding eating when you don't need to because emotions are getting the best of you. The hardest time for me to avoid this kind of eating is at night. If I get bored, or I'm finally relaxing after a long day and my mind has a chance to unwind, I tend to become unfocused. That's the time I seem to get the hungriest. Night time is always a challenge for me, especially if I get bored. Do the best you can to keep your mind from giving its attention to unneeded food.

Food Allergies:

You can have food allergies and not even know it because the symptoms are minor.[3] Sometimes something as simple as bloating can be a sign of a minor food allergy.[3] Gluten is a common ingredient that people are allergic to. People are much more aware of this ingredient than in the days of past, and you will find many food products labeled gluten-free now. The easiest way to find out if you are allergic to a particular kind of food is to simply avoid it for a while to see if the symptoms go away. A food journal is very helpful when checking for food allergies. Major food allergies are usually obvious and can be very dangerous. For your safety, if you suspect you might have food allergies I recommend checking with your doctor and consult him or her about it, especially if you think it may be a major food allergy.

Interesting Fact on Fruits and Vegetables:

Technically speaking, any plant-based food with a seed is considered a fruit.[108] Often, what are thought of as vegetables are actually fruits. A few examples: pumpkins, peas, corn, beans (yes beans), bell peppers, eggplants, cucumbers, squash, and tomatoes are actually fruits![108] However, I would not suggest putting these fruits in a fruit salad as that would be thoroughly disgusting. Vegetables, on the other hand, are all the other non-seeded parts of the plant including the leaves, roots, stems, and even the flower buds, such as broccoli.[108] Now, why do we classify things like beans as vegetables when they are not at all vegetables, but fruit? Quite simple really; taste. Its culinary tradition to classify fruits and veggies based on taste.[108] Fruit are sweet; vegetables are more savory and less sweet. All in all, as interesting as it may be to know this, it doesn't matter, because both fruits and vegetables are essential to your everyday diet. So, eat away.

Corn Myths:

The notion that corn is unhealthy for you is rubbish. Some may scoff at that, but I say it for good reason. I'm willing to bet if you asked almost any registered dietician they would agree with me. There are several false myths about corn. The perception that corn is not good for you more than likely came from the fact that it's high in starch, which is a carbohydrate. Given the fact that our nation is currently going through a carb phobia phase, this is likely the main culprit behind the idea that corn is bad for you. Nothing could be further from the truth. Corn contains nutrients, just as other healthy vegetable options do as well.

For some reason, it's a common notion that corn isn't a good source of nutrients. Corn may not be a superfood with massive amounts of nutritional value, such as the likes of certain other vegetables, but it does bring some nutrients to the table. Corn's nutritional value comes in the form of certain kinds of B vitamins, and vitamin C. Corn also contains magnesium and potassium. More specifically, corn has a couple important antioxidants, zeaxanthin and lutein, which are good for your eyes.[109]

Another strange myth about corn that you can dispel is the thought that you shouldn't eat corn because it's high in sugar. Nonsense. Although corn does have sugar in it, hence the name sweet corn, it doesn't even have as much sugar as other fruits. Let's compare it to a banana. Are bananas considered unhealthy because they contain sugar? No. Then neither should corn be considered unhealthy for the same reason. Corn contains far less sugar than a banana. Both an ear of corn and a banana contain about the same amount of calories, a little over a 100. However, a banana has about 15 grams of sugar, while an ear of corn only has about six to eight grams of sugar.

Finally, another myth that corn has a bad rep for is the fact that many think corn can't be digested. It is true that corn has a good amount of insoluble fiber, but this is a good thing.[109] If you eat too much corn, you may end up seeing some in your stools, but insoluble fiber helps to feed the good bacteria in our intestines. This kind of fiber is what gets stuff moving through the intestines, which is important.[110]

Meal Timing:

I've talked before about not eating too close to bedtime, but you also don't want to eat too close to a workout. It's not a good idea to jump right into a workout after eating; wait at least an hour to an hour and a half to let your stomach settle.[3] First off, you don't want to cramp up. Also, if you eat too close to your workout, you can end up feeling sluggish and turn out a less than stellar performance. Sluggishness can happen because after you eat blood is being sent to your gut to aid in digestion, but working muscles need blood as well when you exercise, so your body is in a battle for blood.[3] This battle is not a pleasant feeling, I'll tell you that. I know, I've made this mistake before. You can even end up getting sick and hurling up your meal if you work out too soon after eating.[3] This is especially true if you've just had a big meal and go right into an intense workout. Also, food is fuel for your workouts. Don't eat like a bird and expect to have an abundance of energy, but of course, don't gorge either.

A Word about Bread:

The carb-phobia that is plaguing this country right now has brought about the idea in many minds that bread is an evil food, and must be avoided if you seek weight loss. Let me tell you this; unless I have a super human body, which is somehow unaffected by the consumption of bread, I can assure you this is false. The most successful weight loss stint I've ever had was a time I lost 41 pounds over the course of several months. At that time, I lost about an average of two pounds a week, which is the ideal amount. During the entire time of my greatest weight loss achievement, I ate bread, and plenty of it. I ate it nearly every day, but I didn't overdo it. I ate bread in moderation. Also, with the exception of a few occasions, I avoided white bread all together. As I've previously mentioned, I recommend avoiding white bread as this is not a healthy option. Other than the case with white bread, the truth of the matter is that you can eat bread if you so choose. However, treat it the same as you would with nearly any other food; eat it in moderation.

Healthy Food Recipes:

An entire book can be written on recipes and specific meal plans, and many are. For simplicity's sake, I do not include any recipes or specific meal plans here as this book is more about blunders to avoid and diet rules to follow that can result in the perfect beach physique. What I do recommend is to use the website I have listed below. This is a terrific site that is free to use and has more than you would ever need regarding healthy recipes or meal plans: http://www.eatingwell.com/

Chapter Twelve Summary:

- **The amount of servings per food group you need in a day are wholly dependent on your needs and goals, and how many calories you are eating in each particular food group.**

- **Knowing serving sizes are important for tracking calories, and remember to use proper portion control.**

- **Remember the rule that a balanced diet is always the best option for your health and waistline.**

- About 45 to 60 percent of your diet should come from calories contained in vegetables, fruits, and grains. Roughly 10 to 35 percent of calories in your diet should come from proteins and the same percentages from healthy fats. You should also include one to two servings of dairy a day.

- Meat: A serving size is roughly the size of a deck of cards, or you can measure in ounces with a food scale (three ounces of cooked meat equals one serving.) Lean meats are the best, turkey being king. White meat contains fewer calories and fat than dark meat. I recommend eating skinless chicken. Eggs are the best source of protein because they contain amino acids needed to utilize the protein. I recommend fish like salmon, tilapia, and tuna; these are a good source of brain healthy omega-3 fatty acids, and fish is also a good source of protein.

- Most veggies retain vitamins and minerals the best when steaming them rather than boiling them. Boiling can cause vitamin and mineral leaching. Eating them raw is another healthy option. A serving size is about the size of a fist.

- Eat more veggies than fruits, but fruits are a great snack you can eat abundantly. One serving size of fruit is approximately the size of a baseball.

- Eat grains in moderation, and it's best to eat whole grains. Limit or don't eat any refined grains from things like breakfast cereals, or white bread. One serving is about ½ the size of a baseball.

- Healthy fats come from things like dairy, yogurt, avocados, etc. I recommend going light on dairy, including milk (one cup = one serving) and cheese (1 and ½ ounces is one serving). These have nutritional value and health benefits, but tend to be high in calories and fat, and can slow up the digestive system. A teaspoon is one serving of fats or oils, which is about the size of the tip of your thumb.

- The three primary macronutrients are fats, carbs, and protein. One gram of fat is equal to nine calories. Carbs and protein are four calories per gram.

- Cooking methods: limit frying or simply throw the fryer out, as this adds tons of calories and fat. Baking is better than frying because you don't need to add fats and calories from cooking oil. Other healthy cooking methods are steaming, boiling, microwaving, poaching, broiling, grilling, or stir-frying. There are lots of other methods, but the ones listed are the ones I recommend as the healthiest.

- Ingredient labels list the order of ingredients from the most to the least by weight, so if the first ingredient is sugar, that's what the food is mostly made of. Although difficult with American food, avoid food with ingredients you don't know or can't pronounce; these are usually unhealthy.

- Although more expensive than regular food, buy organic if your budget permits you. Better yet, the wisest choice would be to invest the time and energy in starting your own garden.

- Carb Heaven: A term I like to use for tasty but unhealthy foods loaded with simple carbs, or top heavy with carbs such as baked goods or pizza. Don't be fooled by Carb Heaven; it's your health's road to hell.

- In general, I feel that supplements are a waste of money unless you are a professional body builder or something similar. Although they aren't bad for you, so to speak, if you are eating a proper and balanced diet, the average person should never need to spend money on supplements.

- Salt is needed in the body, but not more than 2300 milligrams a day. Too much can cause health problems such as high blood pressure.

- Pepper is good for your heart. Pepper and other natural spices used for flavor can be applied to food generously.

- Although it's perceived that sea salt is healthier for you than regular table salt, they both have roughly the same nutritional value and sodium content. The main differences are taste, texture, and processing. Sea salt is not as processed, which leaves some trace minerals that add taste. Table salt, which comes from underground salt deposits, is more refined and has an additive to help prevent clumping, as well as other unhealthy additives.

- Pink Himalayan salt is a great alternative to regular salt. It's the cleanest and purest salt on earth with many health benefits.

This salt contains over 84 minerals and trace elements and contains far less sodium than regular salt. It's a superior, healthier choice for salt.

- A set of six pack abs will only come with massive determination and continued dieting and exercise. Men have to be below 10 percent body fat, women below 13 percent. These are generalized figures as everyone's body is slightly different and may require more or less body fat removal.

- You can't spot-reduce fat, meaning you can't pick and choose where you want your body to burn fat. You can't just do a bunch of sit-ups and expect belly fat to burn off. Your body will burn fat in accordance with its genetic makeup, and generally, the gut is the last to go because typically most fat is stored there.

- Eat a balanced diet that includes variety. This will ensure you are obtaining a variety of necessary minerals and vitamins.

- When choosing which fruits and veggies to eat, "eat the rainbow." This term means to eat different colored foods, which assures you that you're getting different kinds of vitamins and minerals you need. The color of a fruit or vegetable is indicative of it being abundant in a particular vitamin.

- Not only can unhealthy eating lead to disease, but so can the absence of healthy foods in your diet, like fruits and veggies. They are both good for the waistline, and they're health boosters.

- Dressings on foods, such as ranch, are easily overdone and add lots of calories to food otherwise typically low on calories. One exception is mustard, which quite literally has zero calories.

- If you are a vegetarian, make sure you get plenty of protein from non-meat foods such as nuts, beans, spinach, etc.

- Regular potatoes and sweet potatoes are both healthy choices. It's best to eat them with the skin, for their nutrients. If you skin them do it thinly because most of the nutrients are close to the skin.

- Brown rice is much better for you than white rice. Brown rice is a whole grain with the nutrients intact. White rice is stripped of their nutritious parts during processing, rendering them "empty calories."

- Smart Balance cooking spray is a smarter (no pun intended) choice than regular spray or oil. It has less calories and has a greater nutritional value. Smart Balance butter is a superior choice to regular butter or margarine as well. It's lower in calories and bad fats and has healthy omega-3 fats.

- Cheese should be eaten in moderation. It is a good source of protein and other nutrients, but it tends to be high in calories and fat. Avoid or limit cheese products, which is anything that is less than 51 percent cheese.

- Healthy cheese options: cottage cheese (good source of protein), swiss, parmesan, string cheese, full-fat cheese, and feta.

- Unhealthy cheese options are cheese products, or anything labeled "reduced" this or that. A good rule of thumb to remember is anything that has had naturally occurring ingredients stripped, and others added in their place, is unhealthy for you. Typically the additives food manufacturers use to supplement for lost taste are harmful products.

- Both frozen yogurt and ice cream are loaded to the hills with sugar, but if it's time for that once in a while cheat, opt for frozen yogurt. Typically, frozen yogurt has less sugar and has live and active cultures. If you must have ice cream though, opt for slow churned ice cream, which is lower in fat and still taste as good as regular ice cream.

- Pudding, along with ice cream or frozen yogurt, is one of my favorite occasional cheats. You will have your own favorite cheats of course, but believe it or not you can enjoy the foods you love on occasion and still meet your health and diet goals. However, always remember to indulge in cheats sparingly.

- Emotional eating is a challenge many of us face, and it can be linked to all kinds of health problems because it frequently leads to overeating. Eat with your head, not your emotions. Easier said than done, but the best way to avoid emotional eating is to distract your mind to help focus on something else other than food. Exercise is great for this, especially cardio, which is known to reduce appetite. Strength training or lifting weights can have the opposite effect.

- Food allergies can be minor and difficult to detect, but they can give you simple symptoms such as bloating. The easiest way to find out if you have allergies is to avoid certain foods and see how you feel over time. Keeping a food journal is helpful with this. Seek advice from a doctor if you think you have food allergies, especially a major food allergy, which can be dangerous and sometimes life-threatening.

- Even though culinary tradition categorizes veggies and fruits based on taste (fruits are sweet, vegetables are savory and less sweet), many foods thought to be vegetables are actually fruits. Some examples are beans, cucumbers, and tomatoes.

- Any plant-based food with a seed is a fruit. Vegetables are all the other non-seeded parts of the plant, including the leaves, stems, roots, and even the flower buds, such as broccoli.

- Disregard the notion that corn is bad for you; it is not. There are several false myths about corn, including it being considered unhealthy, it isn't a good source of nutrients, it's high in sugar, and it can't be digested. These are all false myths. Corn is a healthy option just like other vegetables.

- Wait at least an hour to an hour and a half before exercising if you just ate, especially if it was a heavy meal. Ignore this, and you will feel sluggish, have poor performance, and it can even make you sick and hurl up your meal.

- Bread is not an evil food you cannot consume if you desire weight loss. During my greatest weight loss stint of 41 pounds I ate bread nearly every day. However, as I previously mentioned, avoid white bread as this is not a healthy option. Eat other kinds of bread in moderation as you would with nearly any food.

- For healthy recipes and meal plans I recommend using this free site: http://www.eatingwell.com/

Final Thoughts:

Remember this; in general, the basic rules of dieting that have worked in the past still work today. The human race has not evolved, or at least not to the point that the same basic diet rules that worked in the past just suddenly won't work anymore. People tend to overthink things. I know I'm guilty of this; but never forget the basics, they are the foundation. Knowledge about food and its effects on the human body is ever increasing, but most of the basic understandings we already know about dieting haven't seemed to change much, if at all. Theories come and go, but for the most part, the basics have stayed true. Now, with that in mind, I have pointed out in this book that food can have a profound impact on your life, good or bad.

Every single piece of food or drink you choose to put in your mouth will generally have one of two major effects on your body. Food and fluids will either work towards disease over time, or it will fight against it. Food is either your medicine or poison, so choose wisely. Unhealthy foods are what I consider a slow poison to our bodies. These foods are, in part, man's fault for messing with our food's natural state and processing it for mass consumption. Food has a much bigger impact on our lives and health than we give it credit for.

Food is important to how you look, and of course your health. The repercussions of food choices do not happen overnight. It can help sustain you and keep you healthy, or it can slowly kill you with disease and poor health. Here is some food for thought; indulging your cravings for junk food by grabbing that Snickers bar isn't going to have any serious immediate effects, but imagine if horrible foods like that instantly gave you a nasty deadly disease, or it made you age terribly fast. How fast do you think people would suddenly change their diets if the adverse effects of poor food choices had an immediate impact? I'm thinking pretty damn quickly. Junk food would not sell, and food manufacturers would have to focus entirely on wholesome, healthy food products.

Imagine if food had to be labeled by the potential diseases they can cause over time. This would, without a doubt, make people rethink their food buying habits. In fact, think about it this way, if cigarettes have a Surgeon General's warning that they can cause cancer and all kinds of other horrible health issues, including pregnancy complications, then why can't unhealthy foods be labeled the same way? That may sound extreme and will likely never happen because of food manufacturers' enormous power, but I do believe it would certainly change the overall health of this country, and the world. Imagine also if we could rename foods for what they may cause if you eat them too much overtime; cheesecake changes to cancer, Little Debbie snacks to little diabetes snacks. Ice cream: high blood pressure. A steak full of saturated fat: heart attack. Cake: cellulite, etc. I think you'd be seeing poor food choices disappear from shelves in stores across the country pretty quickly.

However, because our bodies are so resilient, it can take years of abusing your body with junk food to have any serious, regretful consequences.

Therefore you won't see food labels like the ones I've discussed, because it would put too many companies out of business. Greed and power have its claws spread out all throughout society here in America, and many other parts of the world. Keep in mind, it is a fact that unhealthy foods can have the same slow effect on our bodies in a similar manner as cigarettes do.[111]

Except for the lucky ones that seem to have indestructible bodies, never develop cancer, and live to be a 100 years old or better, cigarettes will slowly kill you. Having one cigarette won't kill you, but smoking pack after pack can eventually catch up to you over time. However, when it comes to food, I can assure you it is ok to cheat and indulge in some junk food now and again. Eating junk food sparingly will have little to no effect on your long-term health or body composition; but go light on the crap food. When you eat junk food and sweets excessively over an extended period of time is when it becomes extremely risky for your health. This is how developing disease, and even potentially dying young, can occur. I want you to be healthy and to enjoy life for as long as possible. Because I am a lover of people, this is what I want for everyone.

You see, we are a very reactive country when it comes to our health. We should be more proactive and worry much more significantly about prevention of disease than we currently do, rather than waiting until disease arrives to do anything about it. Being more proactive would have the potential to save the U.S. billions in healthcare costs each year. You would think our government would have a vested interest in our health, considering how much is paid out in Medicare costs each year; but that is a whole other book to write about. To switch gears, and with that being said, the time to start your new diet plan or to follow the advice I've laid out in this book is right now.

When starting something new, or changing your ways, you should always think to yourself; today is Monday. Everyone wants to start fresh on Monday. "I'll do this Monday." "I'm going to start working out again on Monday." How many times have you heard that, or maybe said it yourself? Hell,

I've done it. Guilty! That's the wrong approach. Every day is a new day. Your Monday can be whatever day you want it to be. Mondays do not suck, they are a day of refresh, and everything starts anew.

One of the good things about the advice in this book is the fact that you don't need to go out and spend extra money on a gym membership to apply the advice, if you don't want to. Healthy food may not be cheap, but it doesn't cost you anything extra to implement the diet rules I've laid out for you in this book. Although I will say, I am a very strong advocate for the gym, or at least working out at home (or wherever you possibly can), and for health reasons alone you need to exercise. Do not neglect your fitness just because you diet well. Working out at home just using body weight exercises, is free if you choose not to purchase a gym membership.

Here are some last few pieces of advice when it comes to making the right food choices. Ultimately, the purpose of food is to give us energy and to keep us alive. Food is not on this planet for the sole intention of providing pleasure. We should all be eating to survive and thrive, but not living to eat. A good rule to follow, if you want to eat right and avoid processed garbage, is this; if it doesn't swim in the water, fly in the sky, run on the ground, or grow in the ground, don't eat it.

If you eat like crap, you are slowly killing yourself. Some may argue that you are going to die anyway, so why not just enjoy the foods and your life the way you want? Yes, it's true we will all die someday. However, what's your quality of life going to be like if you fall ill to disease at a young age, or feel like crap most of the time because you eat like crap? Do you want a body worthy of the beach, or to be scared of the mirror? I am in no way saying that to engage in "fat shaming", however, you can't expect optimal health and to look your best if you don't eat right and take care of yourself. A lot of times, looking and feeling like crap directly coincides with poor eating choices. That's what I like to call "health shaming", and I have no problem dishing it out because this country needs a wake-up call when it comes to health and food. Eating healthy can make you feel good, and life is better when you feel good. That's truth. I say yes, enjoy the one life you have and the occasional treat, but realize that enjoying just any old thing you want, just for the sake of pleasure, whether it be food related or not, may have consequences that later produce regret.

Finally, I leave you with these final thoughts. The choices we make can have a profound and lasting, or even permanent, effect on our lives. We all make mistakes, and the best thing to do when you make a mistake is to not condemn yourself from falling short of perfection, but to use it as a learning experience to help correct your ways. I will also tell you that it is easier to make better choices when you concern yourself with what really matters in life. My advice to you is to worry less about buying the newest iPhone or tech gadget and instead redirect some extra funds you may have on healthy, organic foods. Worry more about what is going into your body (and your health) than staying up to date on the latest and greatest tech devices, or keeping up with the Jones's. Finally, it is my hope that this book will be the go-to nutritional guide that you can refer to any time you need to remember a diet rule and want to stay on top of your game to achieve the best results possible, and remain blunder free in the kitchen. Good luck and good health to you.

About the Author:
Marshall Nash

A Maine resident his whole life, Marshall Nash grew up in the small town of Pittsfield Maine. He spent much of his youth playing sports, learning the art of bodybuilding, and becoming a student of health and nutrition. Sports, health, and fitness have always been his number one passion, which subsequently drove him down a path to become a nationally certified personal fitness trainer and a nutritional coach.

Through the years, Marshall has collected a massive volume of knowledge on the subject of health, fitness, and diet. His mission is to share as much of that knowledge as possible with the world and to educate as many as he can on not only what to do, but also on the avoidable mistakes that are made time and time again that hold individuals back from attaining their diet and fitness goals. Marshall is a devoted father of two; daughter Kenzie and son

Mikie. He has many interests that extend beyond health, fitness, and nutrition; one of them is spending time with his children, family, and friends. A lover of people, Marshall continues to educate people through consultations and is in hopes of being an inspiration for what can be accomplished through willpower and dedication to one's goals in life.

One More Thing:

Thank you for taking the time to read **Blunders In The Kitchen: Diet Mistakes to Avoid While Fueling the Perfect Beach Physique.** If you enjoyed this book and found it to be useful for you, I would be very grateful if you would post a review on Amazon. Your support and feedback are truly appreciated, and it certainly does make a difference. I take the time to personally read all of the reviews so I can get your feedback and make this book the absolute best it can possibly be.

If you would like to leave a review for this book, then you can simply visit the link below. Thank you so much for your support!

https://www.amazon.com/review/create-review/ref=cm_cr_dp_d_wr_but_btm?ie=UTF8&channel=glance-detail&asin=B073NN8H5H#

Other Books by Marshall A. Nash:

Blunders In The Gym: Fitness Mistakes to Avoid for Physique Perfection

Connect with Marshall A. Nash:

Thank you so much for taking the time to read this book. It is a blessing to be able to be your coach through this book. I'm excited for what the knowledge in this book can do for your health and physique, and for what it can do to help you reach your goals and remain blunder free.

Any questions? Contact me here I'm glad to help!: mailto: Marshallnashauthor@gmail.com

You can follow me on Twitter: @MrMarshallNash

You can also connect with me on Facebook here: https://www.facebook.com/MarshallANash/

I wish you the best of health, happiness, and success in reaching your goals!

Yours' In Health,

Marshall A. Nash

Notes

References:

1. Cespedes, Andrea. "What Happens If You Overstuff Your Stomach?"
   LIVESTRONG.COM. July 18, 2017. Accessed January 27, 2018.
   https://www.livestrong.com/article/450521-what-happens-if-i-
   overstuffed-my-stomach/.

2. Styles, Serena. "How to Know When Your Stomach Is Full & to Stop
   Eating?" Healthy Eating | SF Gate. March 31, 2018. Accessed October 31,
   2018. http://healthyeating.sfgate.com/stomach-full-stop-eating-
   3080.html.

3. Deane, Lisa. "Nutrition, Flexibility, Cardiovasular." Personal Fitness Trainer
   National Certification Course by World Instructor Training Schools from
   Kennebec Valley Community College, Fairfield, ME, March 31, 2012.

4. Hynd, Rachel. "Fasting Has Many Benefits for the Body."
   Chicagotribune.com. February 24, 2015. Accessed February 04, 2018.
   https://www.chicagotribune.com/lifestyles/health/sns-green-effective-
   fasting-benfits-story.html.

5. Patz, Aviva. "20 Signs You're Too Obsessed With Your Weight ."
   Health.com. 2018. Accessed February 04, 2018.
   https://www.health.com/health/gallery/0,,20983085,00.html#you-ve-
   lost-your-other-passions-0

6. Smith, Jessica. "When Your Weight Fluctuates: What's Normal and What's
   Not." Shape.com. December 17, 2015. Accessed February 04, 2018.
   https://www.shape.com/lifestyle/mind-and-body/when-your-weight-
   fluctuates-whats-normal-and-whats-not.

7. Schwarzenegger, Arnold, and Bill Dobbins. "A Summary Of Fat-Loss Diet
   Rules." In *The New Encyclopedia of Modern Bodybuilding*, 746. New
   York, NY: Simon & Schuster, 1998.

8. Mayo Clinic Staff. "Metabolism and Weight Loss: How You Burn Calories."
   Mayo Clinic. August 30, 2017. Accessed October 29, 2018.
   https://www.mayoclinic.org/healthy-lifestyle/weight-loss/in-
   depth/metabolism/art-20046508.

9. Kent, Linda Tarr. "A Pound of Fat Vs. a Pound of Muscle."
   LIVESTRONG.COM. September 11, 2017. Accessed February 06, 2018.

https://www.livestrong.com/article/438693-a-pound-of-fat-vs-a-pound-of-muscle/.

10. Scott, Jennifer R. "Body Composition and Body Fat Percent." Verywell Fit. May 09, 2018. Accessed October 29, 2018. https://www.verywellfit.com/what-is-body-composition-3495614.

11. Blokker, Shaun. 2013. "Having a Hard Time Losing Weight with INSANITY?"Youtube vide, 3:58. Published March 17, 2013. Accessed: Febuary 06, 2018. https://www.youtube.com/watch?v=DNdCGW5fJ44

12. George, K. "Important Indications of an Under-Active Thyroid." ActiveBeat. May 09, 2018. Accessed October 29, 2018. https://www.activebeat.co/your-health/8-indications-of-an-under-active-thyroid/4/.

13. Mayo Clinic Staff. "Hypothyroidism (underactive Thyroid)." Mayo Clinic. May 22, 2018. Accessed February 06, 2018. https://www.mayoclinic.org/diseases-conditions/hypothyroidism/symptoms-causes/syc-20350284.

14. Braverman, Jody. "Weight Loss & Starvation Mode." LIVESTRONG.COM. July 18, 2017. Accessed February 10, 2018. https://www.livestrong.com/article/264810-weight-loss-starvation-mode/.

15. Mayo Clinic Staff. "Counting Calories: Get Back to Weight-loss Basics." Mayo Clinic. March 28, 2018. Accessed February 10, 2018. https://www.mayoclinic.org/healthy-lifestyle/weight-loss/in-depth/calories/art-20048065.

16. Dunford, Marie, PhD, RD. "Effect of Metabolic Rate on Energy Balance." In *Fundamentals of Sport and Exercise Nutrition*, 32. Fundamentals of Sport and Exercise Science Series. Champaign, IL: Human Kinetics, 2010

17. Nordqvist, Christian. "How Many Calories Should I Eat a Day?" Medical News Today. February 12, 2018. Accessed October 31, 2018. https://www.medicalnewstoday.com/articles/245588.php.

18. Thompson, Dixie L, PhD, FACSM. "Body Mass Index." In *Fitness Professional's Handbook*, 97. 5th ed. Champaign, IL: Human Kinetics, 2007.

19. Suss, Jessica. "Here's Why Weight Loss Is 80 Percent Diet And 20 Percent Exercise." Simplemost. September 28, 2016. Accessed February 10,

2018. https://www.simplemost.com/weight-loss-80-percent-diet-20-percent-exercise/.

20. Gunnars, Kris, BSc. "Daily Intake of Sugar - How Much Sugar Should You Eat Per Day?" Healthline. June 28, 2018. Accessed October 31, 2018. https://www.healthline.com/nutrition/how-much-sugar-per-day.

21. Peluso, Michael R, PhD. "How to Slow Glucose Absorption." Healthy Eating | SF Gate. June 11, 2018. Accessed October 31, 2018. https://healthyeating.sfgate.com/slow-glucose-absorption-6661.html.

22. Wbur. "Is Sugar More Addictive Than Cocaine?" Wbur. January 07, 2015. Accessed March 04, 2018. http://www.wbur.org/hereandnow/2015/01/07/sugar-health-research.

23. Gunnars, Kris, BSc. "10 Similarities Between Sugar, Junk Food and Abusive Drugs." Healthline. September 23, 2014. Accessed March 04, 2018. https://www.healthline.com/nutrition/10-similarities-between-junk-foods-and-drugs.

24. Gunnars, Kris, BSc. "Daily Intake of Sugar — How Much Sugar Should You Eat Per Day?" Healthline. June 28, 2018. Accessed October 31, 2018. https://www.healthline.com/nutrition/how-much-sugar-per-day#section2

25. UCSF. "Hidden in Plain Sight." SugarScience.UCSF.edu. April 27, 2018. Accessed October 31, 2018. http://sugarscience.ucsf.edu/hidden-in-plain-sight/#.W9n95XtKjIV.

26. Gunnars, Kris, BSc. "Daily Intake of Sugar — How Much Sugar Should You Eat Per Day?" Healthline. June 28, 2018. Accessed November 02, 2018. https://www.healthline.com/nutrition/how-much-sugar-per-day#section3.

27. WebMD. "Low-Fat Diet: Why Fat-Free Isn't Trouble-Free." WebMD. November 05, 2016. Accessed March 04, 2018. https://www.webmd.com/diet/guide/low-fat-diet#1.

28. UCSF. "Hidden in Plain Sight." SugarScience.UCSF.edu. April 27, 2018. Accessed November 02, 2018. http://sugarscience.ucsf.edu/hidden-in-plain-sight/#.W_c-NDhKjIU.

29. Talens, Dick. "The Difference Between Sugar and Sugar Alcohols." Vitals. April 28, 2015. Accessed March 04, 2018. https://vitals.lifehacker.com/the-difference-between-sugar-and-sugar-alcohols-1700561078.

30. Food Insight. "Sugar Alcohols Fact Sheet." FoodInsight.org. October 14, 2009. Accessed November 04, 2018. https://www.foodinsight.org/articles/sugar-alcohols-fact-sheet.

31. McNight, Clay. "Sugar Alcohol & Weight Loss." LIVESTRONG.COM. July 18, 2017. Accessed November 04, 2018. https://www.livestrong.com/article/301215-sugar-alcohol-weight-loss/.

32. Shai, Iris, RD, PhD, et al. "Weight Loss with a Low-Carbohydrate, Mediterranean, or Low-Fat Diet." *New England Journal of Medicine* 359, no. 20 (July 17, 2008): 229-41. Accessed March 11, 2018. doi:10.1056/nejmc081747.

33. Mayo Clinic Staff. "Weight Loss: Gain Control of Emotional Eating." Mayo Clinic. October 03, 2015. Accessed March 11, 2018. https://www.mayoclinic.org/healthy-lifestyle/weight-loss/in-depth/weight-loss/art-20047342.

34. Leproult, Rachel, and Eve Van Cauter, PhD. "Role of Sleep and Sleep Loss in Hormonal Release and Metabolism." *Pediatric Neuroendocrinology Endocrine Development*, November 24, 2009, 11-21. Accessed March 11, 2018. doi:10.1159/000262524.

35. Dunford, Marie, PhD, RD . "What Is Carbohydrate and How Does It Relate to Exercise?" In *Fundamentals of Sport and Exercise Nutrition*, 41. Fundamentals of Sport and Exercise Science Series. Champaign, IL: Human Kinetics, 2010.

36. Reed, Karen. "9 Symptoms of Glucose Intolerance You Should Be Aware Of." Positive Health Wellness. May 30, 2017. Accessed March 11, 2018. https://www.positivehealthwellness.com/diet-nutrition/9-symptoms-glucose-intolerance-aware/.

37. Breus, Michael J, PhD. "Could Lack of Sleep Make You Crave Sweets?" The Oz Blog. January 02, 2014. Accessed March 11, 2018. http://blog.doctoroz.com/oz-experts/could-lack-of-sleep-make-you-crave-sweets.

38. Aronson, Dina, MS, RD. "Cortisol — Its Role in Stress, Inflammation, and Indications for Diet Therapy." *Today's Dietitian*, November 2009, 38. November 2009. Accessed March 11, 2018. https://www.todaysdietitian.com/newarchives/111609p38.shtml.

39. Thompson, Dixie L., PhD, FASCM. "Water." In *Fitness Professional's Handbook*, 110. 5th ed. Champaign, IL: Human Kinetics, 2007.

40. Mundel, Toby, PhD. "Health Check: What Happens to Your Body When You're Dehydrated?" The Conversation. January 31, 2016. Accessed March 11, 2018. https://theconversation.com/health-check-what-happens-to-your-body-when-youre-dehydrated-50462.

41. Health Alkaline. "Drinking Water Before You Get Thirsty." Health Alkaline. January 20, 2015. Accessed March 11, 2018. http://www.healthalkaline.com/drinking-water-before-you-get-thirsty/.

42. Perlman, Howard. "The Water in You." The USGS Water Science School. July 23, 2018. Accessed November 06, 2018. https://water.usgs.gov/edu/propertyyou.html.

43. WebMD. "Causes of Fatigue and Sleepiness and How to Fight Them." WebMD. February 14, 2018. Accessed September 03, 2018. https://www.webmd.com/sleep-disorders/ss/slideshow-fatigue-causes-and-remedies.

44. Gundersen, Melissa. "Hydration – The Key To Good Digestion." Gut Health Project. August 30, 2015. Accessed September 03, 2018. https://www.guthealthproject.com/hydration-the-key-to-good-digestion/.

45. Bright Side. "What Would Happen If You Replace All Drinks with Water." Bright Side. November 06, 2018. Accessed November 06, 2018. https://brightside.me/inspiration-health/what-would-happen-if-you-replace-all-drinks-with-water-315660/.

46. Talk, Earth. "The Dangers of Reusing Plastic Bottles." ThoughtCo. October 29, 2018. Accessed November 08, 2018. https://www.thoughtco.com/reusing-plastic-bottles-serious-health-hazards-1204028.

47. Summers, Joseph. "When You Drink Water On An Empty Stomach After Waking Up, These 8 Amazing Things Will Happen." Lifehack. January 17, 2018. Accessed September 03, 2018. https://www.lifehack.org/449117/when-you-drink-water-on-an-empty-stomach-after-waking-up-these-8-amazing-things-will-happen.

48. Holohan, Meghan. "Should You Drink Warm or Cold Water When You Wake Up? Experts Weigh in." TODAY.com. August 26, 2016. Accessed September 03, 2018. https://www.today.com/health/should-you-drink-warm-or-cold-water-when-you-wake-t51041.

49. BrainWorld. "Brain Basics: Know Your Brain." Brain World. November 02, 2017. Accessed November 08, 2018. https://brainworldmagazine.com/brain-concepts/.

50. Maughan, R.j. "Fluid and Electrolyte Loss and Replacement in Exercise*." *Journal of Sports Sciences* 9, no. Sup1 (November 14, 2007): 117-42. Accessed November 8, 2018. doi:10.1080/02640419108729870.

51. Oberst, Lindsay. "13 Wonderfully Healing Drinks You Should Be Sipping — Especially When You're Sick." Food Revolution Network. February 12, 2018. Accessed September 03, 2018. https://foodrevolution.org/blog/home-remedies-cold-flu-drinks/.

52. Schofield, Kirsten. "7 Natural Remedies for Your Upset Stomach." Healthline. April 14, 2017. Accessed November 8, 2018. https://www.healthline.com/health/digestive-health/natural-upset-stomach-remedies#ginger.

53. Benshosan, April. "Science Says Aspartame Is Worse Than Sugar." Eat This Not That. November 30, 2016. Accessed September 03, 2018. https://www.eatthis.com/aspartame-side-effects/.

54. Zeratsky, Katherine, RD., LD. "I've Been Seeing Ads That Say Caffeinated Drinks Hydrate You as Well as Water Does. Is This True?" Mayo Clinic. September 12, 2017. Accessed September 03, 2018. https://www.mayoclinic.org/healthy-lifestyle/nutrition-and-healthy-eating/expert-answers/caffeinated-drinks/faq-20057965.

55. Nehlig, Astrid, Jean-Luc Daval, and Gérard Debry. "Caffeine and the Central Nervous System: Mechanisms of Action, Biochemical, Metabolic and Psychostimulant Effects." *Brain Research Reviews* 17, no. 2 (March 11, 2003): 139-70. Accessed November 11, 2018. doi:10.1016/0165-0173(92)90012-b.

56. Marcus, Mary Brophy. "Your Daily Coffee Just Might Jolt Your Memory." WebMD. January 12, 2014. Accessed September 03, 2018. https://www.webmd.com/brain/news/20140112/your-daily-coffee-just-might-jolt-your-memory#1.

57. Mayo Clinic Staff. "Hangovers." Mayo Clinic. December 16, 2017. Accessed September 03, 2018. https://www.mayoclinic.org/diseases-conditions/hangovers/symptoms-causes/syc-20373012.

58. Mayo Clinic Staff. "Dietary Fiber: Essential for a Healthy Diet." Mayo Clinic. September 22, 2015. Accessed September 03, 2018.

https://www.mayoclinic.org/healthy-lifestyle/nutrition-and-healthy-eating/in-depth/fiber/art-20043983.

59. Mayo Clinic Staff. "Water: How Much Should You Drink Every Day?" Mayo Clinic. September 06, 2017. Accessed September 03, 2018. https://www.mayoclinic.org/healthy-lifestyle/nutrition-and-healthy-eating/in-depth/water/art-20044256.

60. Milk Composition & Synthesis Resource Library. "Milk Composition - Water." Milk Composition & Synthesis Resource Library. Accessed September 03, 2018. http://ansci.illinois.edu/static/ansc438/Milkcompsynth/milkcomp_water.html.

61. HealthyEating.org. "Nutrients in Milk." HealthyEating.org. Accessed September 03, 2018. https://www.healthyeating.org/Milk-Dairy/Nutrients-in-Milk-Cheese-Yogurt/Nutrients-in-Milk.

62. Reinagel, Monica, MS, LD/N, CNS. "How Much Protein Can the Body Absorb?" Quick and Dirty Tips. July 01, 2015. Accessed September 03, 2018. https://www.quickanddirtytips.com/health-fitness/healthy-eating/know-your-nutrients/how-much-protein-can-the-body-absorb?page=1.

63. Schwarzenegger, Arnold, and Bill Dobbins. "Protein Supplements." In *The New Encyclopedia of Modern Bodybuilding*, 709. New York, NY: Simon & Schuster, 1998.

64. Mayo Clinic Staff. "Binge-eating Disorder." Mayo Clinic. May 05, 2018. Accessed September 04, 2018. https://www.mayoclinic.org/diseases-conditions/binge-eating-disorder/symptoms-causes/syc-20353627.

65. Mayo Clinic Staff. "Chronic Stress Puts Your Health at Risk." Mayo Clinic. April 21, 2016. Accessed September 04, 2018. https://www.mayoclinic.org/healthy-lifestyle/stress-management/in-depth/stress/art-20046037.

66. Spritzler, Franziska, RD, CDE. "7 Tips to Get Into Ketosis." Healthline. November 21, 2016. Accessed November 12, 2018. https://www.healthline.com/nutrition/7-tips-to-get-into-ketosis#section1.

67. Thompson, Dixie L., Phd, FASCM. "Essential Nutrients." In *Fitness Professional's Handbook*, 104. 5th ed. Champaign, IL: Human Kinetics, 2007.

68. O'Connor, Anahad. "The Claim: White Meat Is Healthier Than Dark Meat." The New York Times. November 20, 2007. Accessed September 05, 2018. https://www.nytimes.com/2007/11/20/health/nutrition/20real.html.

69. Schwarzenegger, Arnold, and Bill Dobbins. "Protein." In *The New Encyclopedia of Modern Bodybuilding*, 706-07. New York, NY: Simon & Schuster, 1998.

70. Mayo Clinic. "What Are Omega-3 Fatty Acids from Fish Oil?" Mayo Clinic. August 04, 2016. Accessed September 05, 2018. https://www.mayoclinic.org/what-are-omega-3-fatty-acids-from-fish-oil/art-20232583.

71. Makkieh, Khadejah, RD. "Does Boiling Vegetables Deplete Their Nutritional Value?" Healthy Eating | SF Gate. May 12, 2018. Accessed September 05, 2018. https://healthyeating.sfgate.com/boiling-vegetables-deplete-nutritional-value-1438.html.

72. New World Encyclopedia. "Tuber." New World Encyclopedia. December 21, 2015. Accessed September 05, 2018. http://www.newworldencyclopedia.org/entry/Tuber.

73. Gunnars, Kris, BSc. "12 Proven Health Benefits of Avocado." Healthline. June 29, 2018. Accessed November 14, 2018. https://www.healthline.com/nutrition/12-proven-benefits-of-avocado.

74. Hamblin, James, MD. "How People Came to Believe Blueberries Are the Healthiest Fruit." The Atlantic. November 15, 2017. Accessed September 05, 2018. https://www.theatlantic.com/health/archive/2017/11/blueberries/545840/.

75. Enos, Deborah, CN. "'Superfruits' May Bring Some Health Benefits." Live Science. November 10, 2011. Accessed September 05, 2018. https://www.livescience.com/35968-superfruit-pomegranate-acai-gogi-health-benefits.html.

76. Harvard T.H. Chan. "Whole Grains." Harvard T.H. Chan. Accessed November 14, 2018. https://www.hsph.harvard.edu/nutritionsource/what-should-you-eat/whole-grains/.

77. Webb, Denise, PhD, RD. "The Impact of Whole Grains on Health." *Today's Dietitian*, May 2013, 44. Accessed November 14, 2018. https://www.todaysdietitian.com/newarchives/050113p44.shtml.

78. Cunha, John P., DO, FACOEP. "15 Foods That Cause Constipation." MedicineNet. December 06, 2016. Accessed November 14, 2018. https://www.medicinenet.com/top_foods_that_cause_constipation/article.htm#some_supplements.

79. Semeco, Arlene, MS, RD. "Why Cottage Cheese Is Super Healthy and Nutritious." Healthline. October 04, 2016. Accessed November 14, 2018. https://www.healthline.com/nutrition/cottage-cheese-is-super-healthy

80. Creel, Bridget. "The 4 Unhealthiest Cheeses, and The 5 Best Cheeses." The Daily Meal. August 28, 2015. Accessed November 14, 2018. https://www.thedailymeal.com/healthy-eating/4-unhealthiest-cheeses-and-5-best-cheeses.

81. Ipatenco, Sara, M.A.Ed. "Is Feta Cheese Healthy?" Healthy Eating | SF Gate. March 28, 2018. Accessed November 14, 2018. https://healthyeating.sfgate.com/feta-cheese-healthy-3615.html.

82. Magee, Elaine, MPH, RD. "The Benefits of Yogurt." WebMD. 2008. Accessed November 14, 2018. https://www.webmd.com/food-recipes/features/benefits-yogurt#1.

83. Michaels, Jillian. "MYTH: Egg Yolks Are Bad For You." Jillian Michaels. November 09, 2015. Accessed November 14, 2018. https://www.jillianmichaels.com/blog/food-and-nutrition/myth-egg-yolks-are-bad-you.

84. Mayo Clinic Staff. "Nuts and Your Heart: Eating Nuts for Heart Health." Mayo Clinic. September 15, 2016. Accessed November 14, 2018. https://www.mayoclinic.org/diseases-conditions/heart-disease/in-depth/nuts/art-20046635.

85. Watson, Stephanie. "How Bad for You Are Fried Foods?" WebMD. June 22, 2017. Accessed November 16, 2018. https://www.webmd.com/diet/news/20170622/how-bad-for-you-are-fried-foods.

86. DoveMed. "Is Baking Or Frying Food Healthier?" DoveMed. January 09, 2017. Accessed November 16, 2018. https://www.dovemed.com/healthy-living/wellness-center/baking-or-frying-food-healthier/.

87. Fillion, L., and C. J. K. Henry. "Nutrient Losses and Gains during Frying: A Review." *International Journal of Food Sciences and Nutrition* 49, no. 2 (July 06, 2009): 157-68. Accessed November 16, 2018. doi:10.3109/09637489809089395.

88. Mann, Denise. "Trans Fats: The Science and the Risks." WebMD. January 01, 2006. Accessed November 16, 2018. https://www.webmd.com/diet/features/trans-fats-science-and-risks#1.

89. Harvard Health Publishing. "The Truth about Fats: The Good, the Bad, and the In-between." Harvard Health Publishing. August 13, 2018. Accessed November 16, 2018. https://www.health.harvard.edu/staying-healthy/the-truth-about-fats-bad-and-good.

90. Siegel, Kathryn. "The Healthiest Cooking Methods Explained." Time. February 01, 2013. Accessed November 16, 2018. http://healthland.time.com/2013/02/01/the-healthiest-cooking-methods-explained/.

91. Kiddie, Joy Y., MSc, RD. "What Are Antioxidants?" Teamworks Health Clinic. June 07, 2013. Accessed November 16, 2018. http://teamworkshealth.ca/what-are-antioxidants/.

92. Progressive. "What Are Oxidants, and Why Is Everyone so Anti Them?" Progressive. Accessed November 16, 2018. http://blog.progressivenutritional.com/blog/what-are-oxidants-and-why-is-everyone-so-anti-them.

93. Pham-Huy, Lien Ai, Hua He, and Chuong Pham-Huy. "Free Radicals, Antioxidants in Disease and Health." *International Journal of Biomedical Science* 4, no. 2 (June 2008): 89-96. Accessed November 17, 2018. https://www.ncbi.nlm.nih.gov/pmc/articles/PMC3614697/.

94. Breene, Sophia. "What Are Antioxidants, Really?" Greatist. June 20, 2016. Accessed November 17, 2018. https://greatist.com/health/what-are-antioxidants.

95. U.S. Food & Drug Administration. "Changes to the Nutrition Facts Label." U S Food and Drug Administration. November 02, 2018. Accessed November 17, 2018. https://www.fda.gov/Food/GuidanceRegulation/GuidanceDocumentsRegulatoryInformation/LabelingNutrition/ucm385663.htm.

96. U.S. Food & Drug Administration. "How to Understand and Use the Nutrition Facts Label." U S Food and Drug Administration. January 03, 2018. Accessed November 17, 2018. https://www.fda.gov/food/labelingnutrition/ucm274593.htm.

97. Price, Annie, CHHC. "Pink Himalayan Salt Benefits That Make It Superior to Table Salt." Dr. Axe. January 01, 2017. Accessed November 17, 2018. https://draxe.com/pink-himalayan-salt/.

98. Zeratsky, Katherine, R.D., L.D. "What's the Difference between Sea Salt and Table Salt?" Mayo Clinic. May 04, 2016. Accessed November 17, 2018. https://www.mayoclinic.org/healthy-lifestyle/nutrition-and-healthy-eating/expert-answers/sea-salt/faq-20058512.

99. Danforth Jr, Elliot, and Albert Burger. "The Role of Thyroid Hormones in the Control of Energy Expenditure." *Clinics in Endocrinology and Metabolism* 13, no. 3 (April 10, 2010): 581-95. Accessed November 17, 2018. doi:10.1016/s0300-595x(84)80039-0.

100. Chodosh, Sara. "Here's Why Your Body Stores More Fat in Certain Places." Popular Science. January 12, 2018. Accessed November 17, 2018. https://www.popsci.com/why-fat-goes-to-my-whatever.

101. Caris, E.M. "5 Health Benefits of Black Pepper." All You Can Spice. September 13, 2017. Accessed November 17, 2018. https://allyoucanspice.com/blogs/news/5-health-benefits-of-black-pepper.

102. Minnor, McCall. "Can You Really Target Fat in Specific Areas of the Body?" Aaptiv. Accessed November 17, 2018. https://aaptiv.com/magazine/spot-reduction-fat.

103. Appleby, Maia. "What Are the Benefits of Eating Multiple Colored Fruits & Vegetables?" Healthy Eating | SF Gate. Accessed November 17, 2018. https://healthyeating.sfgate.com/benefits-eating-multiple-colored-fruits-vegetables-4676.html.

104. McDonell, Kayla, RD. "Brown vs White Rice - Which Is Better For Your Health?" Healthline. August 31, 2016. Accessed November 18, 2018. https://www.healthline.com/nutrition/brown-vs-white-rice#section1.

105. Semigran, Rachel. "What Exactly Is American Cheese?" Mental Floss. April 12, 2016. Accessed November 18, 2018. http://mentalfloss.com/article/65003/what-exactly-american-cheese.

106. Seidenberg, Casey. "What Does 'natural Flavors' Really Mean?" The Washington Post. July 25, 2017. Accessed November 18, 2018. https://www.washingtonpost.com/lifestyle/wellness/what-does-natural-flavors-really-mean/2017/07/24/eccdc47e-67f7-11e7-a1d7-9a32c91c6f40_story.html?utm_term=.7b9f1cebc8d5&noredirect=on&utm_term=.563aa8eab5b0.

107. UHN Staff. "Aspartame Side Effects: Recent Research Confirms Reasons for Concern." University Health News. November 07, 2017. Accessed November 18, 2018.

https://universityhealthnews.com/daily/nutrition/aspartame-side-effects-recent-research-confirms-reasons-for-concern/.

108. Boulton, Terynn. "The Difference Between Fruits and Vegetables." Today I Found Out. September 04, 2013. Accessed November 18, 2018. http://www.todayifoundout.com/index.php/2013/09/what-is-the-difference-between-fruits-and-vegetables/.

109. Levy, Jillian, CHHC. " Is Corn Healthy? Surprising Facts About the Nutritional Value of Corn." Dr. Axe. September 01, 2015. Accessed November 18, 2018. https://draxe.com/nutritional-value-of-corn/.

110. Gardner, Amanda. "Soluble and Insoluble Fiber: What's the Difference?" WebMD. July 23, 2015. Accessed November 18, 2018. https://www.webmd.com/diet/features/insoluble-soluble-fiber.

111. Brownell, Kelly D., and Kenneth E. Warner. "The Perils of Ignoring History: Big Tobacco Played Dirty and Millions Died. How Similar Is Big Food?" *The Milbank Quarterly* 87, no. 1 (March 11, 2009): 259-94. Accessed November 18, 2018. doi:10.1111/j.1468-0009.2009.00555.x.

112. Deane, Lisa. "Weight Training, Special Populations, First Aid." Personal Fitness Trainer National Certification Course by World Instructor Training Schools from Kennebec Valley Community College, Fairfield, ME, April 14, 2012.

www.ingramcontent.com/pod-product-compliance
Lightning Source LLC
Chambersburg PA
CBHW030430290526
45786CB00001B/221